CHRONIC MUSCULOSKELETAL INJURIES IN THE WORKPLACE

DON RANNEY, M.D., F.R.C.S.
Associate Professor of Kinesiology
Head, School of Anatomy
University of Waterloo
Waterloo, Ontario, Canada

Illustrated by Alan Ranney

W. B. SAUNDERS COMPANY
A Division of Harcourt Brace & Company

Philadelphia, London, Toronto, Montreal, Sydney, Tokyo

W. B. SAUNDERS COMPANY
A Division of Harcourt Brace & Company

The Curtis Center
Independence Square West
Philadelphia, Pennsylvania 19106

Library of Congress Cataloging-in-Publication Data

Ranney, Don.
    Chronic musculoskeletal injuries in the workplace / Don Ranney.—
1st ed.
        p.   cm.
    ISBN 0–7216–6841–0
    1. Musculoskeletal system—Wounds and injuries.   2. Occupational
diseases.   I. Title.
    [DNLM: 1. Musculoskeletal System—injuries.   2. Occupational
Diseases—etiology.   3. Occupational Diseases—rehabilitation.
4. Chronic Disease.   5. Repetition Strain Injury.   WE 140 R211c
1997]
RD732.R36   1997
617.4'73044—dc20
DNLM/DLC   96-23286

CHRONIC MUSCULOSKELETAL INJURIES
IN THE WORKPLACE   ISBN 0–7216–6841–0

Printed in the United States of America.

Last digit is the print number: 9   8   7   6   5   4   3   2

In the hope that your suffering was not in vain, this book is respectfully dedicated to all injured workers whose physical and psychological problems have been incorrectly diagnosed and improperly treated and whose real suffering has been misunderstood.

CONTRIBUTORS

GABRIELE BAMMER, BSc, PhD
National Centre for Epidemiology and Population Health, Australian
National University, Canberra, Australia
When Experts Disagree

JOHN CHONG, MD, MSc, FRCPC
Medical Director, Centre for Human Performance and Health Promotion,
Sir William Osler Health Institute, Hamilton, Ontario, Canada
Physical Therapy for Physical Problems

BRAD K. GRUNERT, PhD
Associate Professor of Psychology, Medical College of Wisconsin,
Milwaukee, Wisconsin
*Psychological Assessment of Chronic Upper Extremity Disorders; When Chronic
Pain is the Problem*

BENTE R. JENSEN, MSc, PhD
Senior Scientist, National Institute of Occupational Health, Copenhagen,
Denmark
Muscle Pathology With Overuse

BRIAN MARTIN, PhD
Department of Science and Technology Studies, University of Wollongong,
NSW, Australia
When Experts Disagree

ALBERTA PICHÉ, RegN, BScN, COHN(C)
Associate Faculty, Conestoga College; Occupational Health Nurse
Consultant; Occupational Health Associate, Pace Consulting Group, Inc.,
Kitchener, Ontario, Canada
Workplace Management of the Injured Worker

DON RANNEY, MD, FRCS
Associate Professor of Kinesiology, Head, School of Anatomy, University of
Waterloo, Waterloo, Ontario, Canada; Orthopaedic Consultant, Chronic
Pain Management Program, St. Mary's Hospital, Kitchener, Ontario,
Canada
*A Controversial Issue; Pathological and Clinical Basis of Chronic Musculoskeletal
Injuries; Pain Perception; Diagnostic Criteria; Neck and Shoulder, Back and
Buttock; Elbow, Forearm, Wrist, and Hand; Clinical Assessment of Nerves and
Vessels; Mind, Body, Society, and the Workplace Environment*

MICHEL ROSSIGNOL, MD, MSc, FRCPC
Assistant Professor, Department of Epidemiology and Biostatistics, Faculty
of Medicine, McGill University; Deputy Director, Centre for Clinical
Epidemiology and Community Studies, Jewish General Hospital, Montreal,
Quebec, Canada
Establishing a Prognosis for Low Back Problems

GISELA SJØGAARD, PhD, DrMed Sc
Associate Professor, University of Copenhagen; Head, Department of
Physiology, National Institute of Occupational Health, Copenhagen,
Denmark
Muscle Pathology With Overuse

RICHARD WELLS, MEng, PhD
Associate Professor of Kinesiology, Associate Dean for Computing and
Special Projects, Department of Kinesiology, Faculty of Applied Health
Sciences, University of Waterloo, Waterloo, Ontario, Canada
Task Analysis; Work-Relatedness of Musculoskeletal Disorders

FOREWORD

The concept of chronic or repetitive injury in the workplace is not new; it was recognized by Ramazzini in his classic work more than two centuries ago. What, then, prompts the current feverish interest in the topic? I believe that the answer, at least in part, has to do with responsibility and money, and, specifically, whose money and whose responsibility. Prior to the introduction of workers' compensation laws in the later 19th century, it was the workers who took the responsibility for their injuries and paid, both in the form of any medical costs that might be incurred and often by the loss of employment itself, if the impairment proved too great to permit them to continue on the job. Over the past century, there has been a gradual shift in attitude, with the employer and workers' compensation carrier responsible for a greater share of the cost incurred for illnesses and injuries that arise at the workplace.

There seems little controversy at this point with regard to acute injuries and to illnesses that develop exclusively from exposure to toxins present only at the workplace. More recently, some have considered that work itself, under certain special circumstances, might be considered pathogenic. This may seem to fly in the face of the well-known benefits of exercise, but work differs from exercise in that the pace may not be under the control of the participant. Furthermore, we now know that exercise-induced hypertrophy is preceded by exercise-induced injury; the hypertrophy may be considered a healing response. It is well recognized that weekend athletes who exceed their limits may suffer from a variety of injuries ranging from blisters to stress fractures. These injuries are not the result of a single trauma, but represent the accumulated effect of minor injuries, with insufficient time for intervening healing. So it may be with the worker, particularly when the conditions at work do not permit a halt, that symptoms or signs of problems first appear. Indeed, in some cases it almost seems a precondition that there be a lack of control of the workplace by the worker for repetitive trauma injury to occur, if one examines reports of recent "outbreaks" in Australia, the United States, and elsewhere.

Other issues, of course, also play a role, and may cloud the picture. If the type of injuries that one typically sees with repetitive use are the same whether the repetitive use occurs in the workplace or at home, then one is left with the worker's testimony as to where the problem first developed. Clearly, the same issue can occur with an acute injury, such as a laceration, which can also occur outside the workplace. Usually with acute injuries, however, there are other witnesses so that the problem of the worker's word versus the employer's does not arise.

Finally, there is the ever-changing issue of what constitutes an injury. Are symptoms alone sufficient, or are some signs pointing to a specific diagnosis necessary? Many epidemiologic studies have focused on symptoms alone, assuming that they are always associated with a diagnosis. Unfortunately, this is not the case; almost everyone will have symptoms of some ache or another, in some place or another, at some time in the course of a year. Pathologic conditions are also associated with symptoms; however, the difference is that there are some associated physical or laboratory findings that can confirm a specific anatomic focus for the problem. Such is the case with fractures and lacerations most obviously, but also for conditions such as trigger finger, carpal tunnel syndrome, de Quervain's disease, and shoulder impingement syndrome. More difficult are the conditions such as lateral epicondylar pain and tenderness along the paths of various tendons, where swelling may not be a prominent feature and where biopsy may show a nonspecific thickening of tendon sheath or synovium, which may or may not be within the realm one might see in "normal" (i.e., asymptomatic) individuals. Such conditions are not often a therapeutic problem for the clinician, because they are typically self-limited and can be managed with a variety of simple symptomatic measures. They only become a problem when they are also the focus of an adversarial process in which, in order to "win," the worker must certify himself or herself as impaired in some way, and the employer "wins" at the price of alienating an employee or, even worse, the cost of losing an experienced worker together with the additional cost of training a replacement. For other problems, are there really no signs, or are we just not (yet) clever enough to find them? When there are signs, how can we be sure we have not been too clever in producing them?

Managing this complex web takes skill, and not the skill likely to be possessed by a single individual. I believe a team approach is best—ideally, a team that includes worker, employer, and medical professionals from a variety of disciplines. Such a group working together is in the best position to determine whether a problem fits more into the realm of the aches and pains of daily life, is exclusively associated with the workplace, or is something in between. This book reviews the current understanding of the pathophysiology, epidemiology, clinical diagnosis, and treatment of work-related injuries. These are the building blocks for a coherent approach to the issue of chronic musculoskeletal injuries in the workplace. One can use the same broad background to formulate the next set of research questions, so that we may understand better the relationship of symptoms to injury or disease, and injury or disease to the worker and the workplace.

PETER AMADIO, MD
President-Elect
American Association of Hand Surgeons

PREFACE

The writing of this book began a few years ago as several invited lectures to occupational health nurses on how to diagnose and treat chronic musculoskeletal injuries that are apparently work related. I was advised then to put my thoughts in print and did so to a limited degree in journal articles. The need to publish more material became apparent with the realization that, after all these years, very few of those individuals responsible for reporting work injuries know how to identify injured structures or even how to determine whether such injuries are work related.

My earlier work in reconstructive hand surgery, followed by two decades of teaching anatomy and sports medicine, had led to the development of a meticulous, anatomically based examination technique that I find useful in my clinical practice. This rarely leaves any doubt about the identity of painful structures, but why are they often painful so long after exposure to trauma?

Part of the answer, at least for muscle, can be found in the chemistry of fatigue and in the structural alterations within the muscle, as described in Chapter 3. Much of the rest of the answer lies in our recent increase in understanding of how chronic pain can cause maladaptative central nervous system responses, some of which have been discovered to be associated with structural changes. Beyond this, there are psychological and sociological factors that are just now be-

coming the focus of attention for many of the health care professionals treating work-related injuries. Unfortunately, there are many who
do not know about these things, and even some who seemingly do
not wish to know.

There have been several excellent textbooks published about work-
related musculoskeletal injuries, whose only fault may be their com-
prehensiveness. This book aims to be smaller, more comfortable, and
more user friendly. Its objective is to provide perspective and promote
understanding, both of which will be of practical value for the "gatekeepers" in occupational medicine.

ACKNOWLEDGMENTS

The identification and management of work-related injuries requires a team approach. The same is true when a book is written on this subject. Writing this book could not have been accomplished without the eager and expert assistance of my collaborators. Beyond these, my greatest thanks goes to my secretary, Janet Coulter, who, as always, accepted with a smile the many almost illegible scrawls I submitted to her. No doubt the keyboarding required contributed to her work-related wrist problem.

To my proofreaders I owe a great debt of gratitude. Each has expertise related to particular aspects of the material presented. These are Hugh Scoggan, senior lab demonstrator in anatomy; Gayle Shellard, secretary and recipient of carpal tunnel surgery; and Elizabeth Valenta, consultant, occupational health nursing.

Because each picture is worth a thousand words, it would take several extra chapters to adequately thank my son Alan for the hand-drawn illustrations he so beautifully produced with the help of his models, Mary and David Blondé and Colleen Moggy.

Finally, I would like to thank, for their encouragement and advice, my colleagues and friends Donald Faithfull, Damien Ireland, Hunter Fry, Sidney Blair, Ed Beharry, Bob Kilborn, Larry Brawley, and Stu McGill.

CONTENTS

1
A Controversial Issue

When a bone is broken at work or a worker's fingers have been amputated, the nature of the injury and its work relatedness are readily apparent. But when a claim is made that repetitive subthreshold stress has injured soft tissue, a number of legitimate questions may be raised. Is there really an injury here or just a perception of injury? To what extent does the pain of injury reflect the seriousness of the problem? What are the contributions of psychological and social factors in pain perception? Is the injury in fact work related: totally, partially, or not all? What is the precise tissue injured? How should it be treated? How should the psychological and sociological consequences of injury be managed? It is these questions that this book seeks to answer.

Pain is a subjective phenomenon. Disability, to the extent that it is pain related, may also be subjective. It therefore comes as no surprise that claims of disability and resultant requests for compensation will be challenged. On one side of the controversy will be the injured worker and the union, on the other side the employer and the insurance company. Caught uncomfortably somewhere between them will be the health care practitioners. Where does the truth lie? Sometimes this can be a question for Solomon. Getting the media involved rarely if every helps the situation and can often make matters much worse. It was media involvement that helped raise the controversy to fever pitch in Australia, and an epidemic of repetitive (or repetition) strain injuries (RSIs) swept the nation. The fire was eventually put out by

1

a determined effort not to discuss the issue. A moratorium was established in 1987 that for several years prevented publication of articles on RSI in the *Medical Journal of Australia*, and in the same year the Australia Public Service Census ceased publishing records of RSI incidence (Bammer, 1990).

In 1985, the Australian Council of Hand Surgery passed the following resolutions regarding RSI:

The seriousness of the national epidemic in view of the costs to the community is recognized.

A pathologic basis to explain the continuation of symptoms is available in a small proportion of cases only.

The majority of these cases stem from nervous causes and can broadly be characterized as occupational neuroses.

The condition is reversible.

Any changes resulting from the disorder are reversible and can be reversed by exercise and normal use.

RSI should be called the reversible fatigue syndrome.

However, workers continued to be injured and many prominent hand surgeons disagreed with these resolutions. The matter was hotly debated and the resolutions were not passed with unanimous support.

In Australia at present, workers' compensation statistics on the incidence of occupational overuse syndrome are published but this syndrome continues to be defined as it was in the *National Code of Practice for the Prevention and Management of Occupational Overuse Syndrome*:

> Occupational overuse syndrome, also known as Repetition Strain Injury (RSI), is a collective term for a range of conditions characterized by discomfort or persistent pain in muscles, tendons and other soft tissues, with or without physical manifestations. Occupational overuse syndrome is *usually* caused or aggravated by work, and is associated with repetitive movement, sustained or constrained postures and/or forceful movements. Psycho-social factors, including stress in the working environment, may be important in the development of occupational overuse syndrome. (National Occupational Health and Safety Committee, 1990, p. 4, *emphasis added*)

Clearly the above definition allows both physical and even purely psychological problems to be called occupational overuse syndrome. But, how can a painful condition that is thought to be due to physical injury when there is none, be called an "overuse" syndrome? What has been overused? On the one hand, many medical practitioners in Australia are unwilling to accept as work related anything except purely and obviously physical problems (Mullaly and Grigg, 1988). Yet under this official definition a person does not have to have a physical problem to be considered to suffer from occupational overuse syndrome. Has RSI just changed its name to occupational overuse syndrome? Apparently so (Bammer, 1988). On the other hand, is RSI (or cumulative trauma disorder in North America) just a sociopolitical phenomenon, as Ireland (1995) claims?

In Europe and North America, and even in Australia today, the camp is divided between believers and nonbelievers. Each side has its outspoken champions. Epidemiologic studies have looked at the prevalence of work-related problems in various industries in an attempt to settle the issue. Some of these have shown quite conclusively that work-related chronic musculoskeletal disorders are related to risk factor exposure (see Stock, 1991). However, how many of these "disorders" are in fact physical injuries, if the data on which they rest are primarily complaints of pain without objective evidence that would lead to a definitive diagnosis? Can pain be verified objectively?

The central chapters of this book provide a methodology for determining whether, and precisely what, structures have been injured. First, however, it is worthwhile reviewing the evidence that overuse at work *can* cause injury to tissues. We also must consider the extent to which psychological and sociological factors can influence pain perception and our belief about its meaning. Then, when treating, for example, tendinitis, it will be clear that we are treating not merely an injured tendon but a whole person who occupies (at least for that person) an important role in society. To be truly effective, therapy must heal not only the body but also the mind, and effectively deal with any related problems in the family and the working environment.

REFERENCES

Bammer G: More than a pain in the arms: A review of the consequences of developing occupational overuse syndrome. J Occup Health Safety Aust NZ 4:389–397, 1988.

Bammer G: The epidemic is over . . . or is it? Australian Society 9(April): 22–24, 1990.

Ireland DCR: Repetition strain injury: The Australian experience. J Hand Surg 20A(Part 2):S53–S56, 1995.

Mullaly J, Grigg L: RSI: Integrating the major theories. Aust J Psych 40:19–33, 1988.

National Occupational Health and Safety Committee: National Code of Practice for the Prevention and Management of Occupational Overuse Syndrome. Canberra, Australian Government Publishing Service, 1990.

Stock SR: Workplace ergonomic factors and the development of musculoskeletal disorders of the neck and upper limbs: A meta-analysis. Am J Ind Med 19:87–107, 1991.

SCIENTIFIC
BASIS _____

2
Pathological and Clinical Basis of Chronic Musculoskeletal Injuries

One of Murphy's lesser known laws states that, if anything is used to its full potential, something will break. This thought-provoking statement reminds us that all structures have a breaking point. Steel, glass, wood, ceramics, and the like are all able to withstand an amount of stress characteristic of their structure. A high enough force will cause disruption with one application. Lesser forces repeated over time will eventually cause fatigue fracture. The same is true of biologic tissue: bone, ligament, tendon, and so on. Repetitive stresses cause cumulative strain with eventual disruption (Fig. 2–1). In fact, we can only learn how strong any material is by tearing it apart.

Biologic tissues have a distinct advantage over inert physical material: their disruptions can heal. This is most dramatically illustrated in the callus that quickly engulfs the ends of a broken bone. A strong scaffolding of cartilage is quickly thrown up around the fracture site. It becomes rigid by calcification (primary callus) and is then replaced by bone (secondary callus). Now the slower and very careful reconstruction can start as the bone ends are united by bone that looks exactly like the original. The scaffolding is much more slowly removed and, if the bone ends have not been displaced, it is frequently impossible to tell on a radiograph that the fracture ever occurred.

This self-healing process also takes place on a microscopic level when stress insufficient to break a tissue is applied. In 1892, Julius Wolff described this phenomenon in bone, which has since been labeled Wolff's Law: When stress is applied to a bone, it becomes

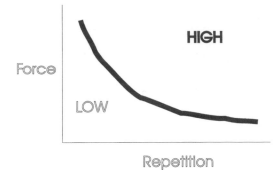

Figure 2–1. Fatigue curve for inert materials and biologic tissues, showing relationship between magnitude of force and the number of repetitions to cause disruption of the tissue.

stronger. A ballerina going *en pointe* (or even *demi-pointe*) takes considerably more stress through her second metatarsal than we do when we walk or even run. Doing this for many hours each day can cause a metatarsal fracture. However, because the stress is applied gradually, instead of the bone breaking, it becomes stronger and noticeably thicker on a radiograph. Thus, graduated stress on bone has promoted increased strength.

The same is true of all tissues. Friction applied repeatedly to the skin stimulates growth of the skin cells. If the cell growth can keep a little ahead of the damage being attempted, the skin becomes thicker and a callus results. Similarly, if one regularly exercises sufficiently, one's heart become larger and stronger. The same applies to muscles elsewhere in the body, as well as to tendons, ligaments, and many other tissues—even the brain. If we use what we have, it becomes stronger; if we do not, it becomes weaker.

However, if the stress applied is greater than the tissue can tolerate, instead of becoming stronger, it breaks down: the skin friction causes a blister or even an ulcer, the muscle is strained, the tendon develops micro-tears, the brain becomes tired, and so on (see Table 2–1). For those problems that affect the musculoskeletal system, the term "repetitive strain injury" (RSI) could legitimately be used, and in Canada this has been the practice. Because these injuries are due to cumulative trauma, Americans and many Canadians prefer the term "cumulative trauma disorder" (CTD). In Japan and Scandinavia, the term "occupational cervico-brachial disorder" has been popular. However, many in Australia are now advocating that this term be applied to work-related complaints that have *no* obvious physical basis. The same trend is developing in America with CTD. In various parts of the world, the term "work-related musculoskeletal disorder" is now becoming popular. Clearly the terminology is confusing! Nerve compression may occur as a result of hypertrophy of tendon synovium or muscles. Such nerve entrapment syndromes are often

TABLE 2–1. Overuse Injuries to Specific Tissues*

Tissue	Types of Injury
Muscle	Tears of muscle tendon junction as a result of high load (eccentric) Fatigue: disruption of muscle substance as a result of static contraction
Tendon	Micro-tears (tendinitis) resulting from high load (the term "peritendinitis" is, in fact, more appropriate because the inflammation is in the surrounding connective tissue) Synovial thickening (tenosynovitis) resulting from friction
Nerve	Hypoxia resulting from compression of blood supply by muscles/tendons

*Adapted by permission from Ranney D: Work-related chronic injuries of the forearm and hand: Their specific diagnosis and management. Ergonomics 36:871–880, 1993.

included under these general terms by some authors, and disputed by others as to whether they belong there. However, the general principle that *tissues can be strained through overuse to the point of injury* is beyond dispute.

A more worthy subject of debate is the *extent* to which physical injury occurs in the workplace, and more particularly whether it is present in a given individual. Psychological stress, boredom, a hostile working environment, lack of job satisfaction, a feeling of loss of control, and the like are increasingly being recognized as playing a large role in both the reporting rate and even the development of such problems. In determining the ability of repetitive activity to injure tissues, we must not forget the psyche and the social setting. However, let us first look at the physical basis for saying these problems can occur.

APPROACHES TO THE STUDY OF REPETITIVE STRAIN INJURY

The approach used in studying the cause of a set of symptoms varies with the condition. Some are amenable to biopsy. Biopsy of a tumor will tell us its nature, and often its seriousness (e.g., whether it is malignant), and sometimes its extent. Another approach is that used by Koch to establish that a particular bacterium was the causative agent for a particular set of symptoms and signs. Koch's postulates state first, that the causative agent could always be found where the disease was present, and, second, that introduction of the causative agent would result in the development of the disease. This is an easy approach when only one causative agent is required, as is often the case with infectious diseases. However, when the problem is attributable to a number of interacting influences (e.g., cardiac atherosclerosis), it may take some time before an appropriate epidemiologic study can be developed that will really explain the pathogenesis.

Biopsy

Biopsies have rarely been performed to investigate presumed overuse injuries. No one would suggest biopsying sprained ankles. The diagnosis is apparent clinically, and a biopsy would only add to the trauma. The same applies to so-called RSI. Given today's adversarial climate between workers, employers, and the compensation system, there is naturally reluctance to ask someone to submit to biopsy just to find out what is going on. However, when surgery is necessary, as for carpal tunnel syndrome, a biopsy is easy to obtain. Of the various studies reported, the most significant has been that of Schuind et al. (1990). They studied histologically 21 cases of idiopathic carpal tunnel syndrome, finding synovial hypertrophy in all. They described the process whereby mechanical stress and tendon friction lead to degenerative changes and fibrous hyperplasia of flexor tendon synovium both in the carpal tunnel and in the digits. Associated trigger finger was found in 29 per cent of cases. Dennett and Fry (1988) biopsied the first dorsal interosseous muscle in 28 women, mostly keyboard operators, who had chronic pain in this muscle as a result of overuse. The pathologic changes found related to severity of symptoms, and some resembled those found in primary fibromyalgia. Chapter 3 of this book discusses muscle pathology in depth as it relates to industrial overuse.

Epidemiologic Studies

Epidemiologic studies have shown that repetitive movement, especially if associated with high force, is more frequently associated with pain and tenderness in the areas concerned than when these same conditions are absent. (A list of these studies is given in the Suggested Reading list at the end of this chapter.) In an excellent review of 54 epidemiologic studies, Stock (1991) reanalyzed the data presented in the three that satisfied her very stringent criteria for statistical analysis. She concluded that specific disorders of tendon and tendon sheath, together with carpal tunnel syndrome, are causally related to repetitive forceful work.

If we accept that overuse injuries can and do occur in industry, how do we know that a particular worker has one? For example, "lateral epicondylitis" may occur in a work environment or be due to sporting activity or household chores. Because of the multifactorial etiology of some problems (e.g., carpal tunnel syndrome), even in a large epidemiologic study, the findings must be viewed with caution. Furthermore, pain, tenderness, numbness, and tingling are very subjective complaints. More objective criteria are needed to satisfy the critics, including this author.

Physiologic Studies

Delayed muscle soreness, muscle swelling, and edema (Asmussen, 1956) and elevated serum levels of muscle enzymes (Nuttal and Jones, 1968) have long been recognized in association with overuse. More recently, muscle blood flow has been found to be reduced by repetitive work in patients diagnosed as having RSI, rather than being increased, as it is in normal subjects (McLean et al., 1988). Recent studies on vascular and metabolic changes in muscle with activity are presented in Chapter 3.

Repeated eccentric (lengthening) contractions are apt to result in injury, as indicated by an increase in the blood inorganic phosphate to phosphocreatinine ratio. Sixty eccentric contractions of wrist flexor muscles in 10 minutes in five normal subjects were enough to induce changes comparable to those at rest in seven patients with destructive muscle disorders (McCully et al., 1988). The most recent data on muscle changes with overuse are presented in Chapter 3. Finally, in the world's largest physiologic laboratory, the sports arena, athletes of the world have noted muscle and tendon strains, tenosynovitis, and nerve entrapment syndrome resulting from overuse for the past several decades. Now industrial athletes complain of similar problems.

LESSONS FROM THE SPORTS MEDICINE MODEL

The clinical basis of chronic musculoskeletal injuries resulting from overuse is well established through experience with athletes. Highly motivated individuals who try to deny their problems and "play through the pain" are stopped short of achieving their objectives by disabling pain with no hope of compensation. These cases demonstrate several points of importance regarding similar injuries diagnosed in an industrial setting:

1. There is an upper limit of stress to which muscles, tendons, bone, skin, and other tissues can be subjected, and beyond which injury will occur.

2. This limit varies greatly from one individual to another and can be greatly influenced by general physical conditioning, body type, and previous trauma.

3. Some people have bodies that can never be made suitable for what they are attempting.

4. Technique of performance may be as important as force and repetition in the pathogenesis of injury.

5. The onset and severity of symptoms relate not only to the severity of the problem but also to the individual's goals and degree of motivation.

6. There are a number of well-defined medical conditions typically found in particular situations, and these are verifiable by clinical tests. Vague pain and generalized aching do not occur. Delayed muscle soreness may occur, and it is in the muscles that have been overused by the activity.

7. Laboratory tests may be valuable but are not regularly required.

8. Treatment is difficult if delayed; rest and modified activity are a vital part of any treatment. Later, strengthening exercises must be done but in a graduated program that does not increase injury.

9. In emotionally charged situations, psychotherapy plays a crucial role in treatment.

Clearly, injuries resulting from repetitive overuse do occur in athletes, and what is too much for one person is not so for another. The same should be true for workers in industry. However, there are differences, as shown in Table 2–2. The greatest of these may be motivation. Most workers are highly motivated, and where compensation for working (psychological as well as financial) exceeds that for not working, that motivation is guaranteed.

One problem caused by ever-increasing technology is that of boredom. It may not be so much that repetitive motion causes tissue damage, but rather that boredom allow us to focus on small, even normal, stress-induced signals from our own bodies. Then, if we have heard that RSI can cause permanent disability, we could even interpret normal fatigue as a sign of impending disaster. The first task of the health care practitioner is to determine whether such fears are to some degree justified. If so, then, to prevent such disaster, one must analyze the problem, arrange treatment, and take appropriate preventative steps.

TABLE 2–2. Comparison of Tennis Elbow Overuse Injury in Athletes and Workers*

	AMATEUR ATHLETE	INDUSTRIAL WORKER
Type of injury	Tendon strain	Tendon strain
Cause	Overuse	Overuse
Principles of treatment	Ice, rest	Ice, rest
	Stretch/strengthen	Stretch/strengthen
	Anti-inflammatories	Anti-inflammatories
Purpose of activity	Enjoyment	Survival
Goals	Excellent performance	Salary mostly
Pressure to continue	Self-esteem	Financial necessity

*Reprinted by permission from Ranney DA: Pain at Work and What to Do About It. Waterloo, Canada, University of Waterloo Press, 1990.

REFERENCES

Asmussen E: Observations on experimental muscle soreness. Acta Rheumatol Scand 2:109–116, 1956.

Dennett X, Fry HJH: Overuse syndrome: A muscle biopsy study. Lancet i: 905–908, 1988.

McCully KK, Argov Z, Boden BP, et al: Detection of muscle injury in humans with 31-P magnetic resonance spectroscopy. Muscle Nerve 11:212–216, 1988.

McLean R, Henke P, Smart R, et al: Blood flow study in patients with RSI syndrome. In Proceedings of the Golden Jubilee Meeting of the Royal Australian College of Physicians, Sydney, May 8–13, 1988, p 497.

Mullaly J, Grigg L: RSI Integrating the major theories. Aust J Psych 40:19–33, 1988.

Nuttal FQ, Jones B: Creatinine kinase and glutamic oxalacetic transaminase activity in serum: Kinetics of change with exercise and effect of physical conditioning. J Lab Clin Med 71:847–854, 1968.

Schuind F, Ventura M, Pasteels JL: Idiopathic carpal tunnel syndrome: Histologic study of flexor tendon synovium. J Hand Surg 15A:497–503, 1990.

Stock SR: Workplace ergonomic factors and the development of musculoskeletal disorders of the neck and upper limbs: A meta-analysis. Am J Ind Med 19:87–107, 1991.

Wolff J: The Law of Bone Remodelling (Maquel P, Furling R, trans). New York, Springer-Verlag, 1986. (originally published in 1892)

SUGGESTED READING: EPIDEMIOLOGICAL STUDIES

Aaras A, Westgaard RH: Further studies of postural load and musculoskeletal injuries of workers at an electro-mechanical assembly plant. Appl Ergonomics 18:211–219, 1987.

Anderson JAD: Shoulder pain and tension neck and their relation to work. Scand J Work Environ Health 10:435–442, 1984.

Armstrong TJ: Ergonomics and cumulative trauma disorders. Hand Clin 2: 553–565, 1986.

Armstrong TJ, Fine LJ, Goldstein SA, et al: Ergonomics considerations in hand and wrist tendinitis. J Hand Surg 12A:830–837, 1987.

Armstrong TJ, Silverstein BA: Upper extremity pain in the workplace—role of usage in causality. In Hadler NM (ed): Clinical Concepts in Regional Musculoskeletal Illness. New York, Grune & Stratton, 1987, pp 333–354.

Dimberg L: The prevalence and causation of tennis elbow (lateral humeral epicondylitis) in a population of workers in an engineering industry. Ergonomics 30:573–580, 1987.

Falck B, Aarnio P: Left-sided carpal tunnel syndrome in butchers. Scan J Work Environ Health 9:291–297, 1983.

Feldman RG, Goldman R, Keyserling WM: Peripheral nerve entrapment syndromes and ergonomic factors. Am J Ind Med 4:661–681, 1983.

Ferguson D: An Australian study of telegraphists' cramp. Br Med Jr 28:280–285, 1971.

Ferguson D: Posture, aching and body build in telephonists. J Hum Ergol 5: 183–186, 1976.

Hagberg M: Occupational musculoskeletal stress and disorders of the neck and shoulder: A review of possible pathophysiology. Int Arch Occup Environ Health 53:269–278, 1984.

Hagberg M, Wegman DH: Prevalence rates and odds ratio of shoulder-neck diseases in different occupational groups. Br J Ind Med 44:610–620, 1987.

Herberts P, Kadefors R: A study of painful shoulder in welders. Acta Orthop Scand 47:381–387, 1976.

Herberts P, Kadefors R, Hogfors C, et al: Shoulder pain and heavy manual work. Clin Orthop 191:166–178, 1984.

Hymovich L, Lindholm M: Hand, wrist and forearm injuries. J Occup Med 8:573–577, 1966.

Ketola R, Konni U: Prevalence of epicondylitis and elbow pain in the meat-processing industry. Scand J Work Environ Health 17:38–54, 1991.

Kuorinka I, Koskinen P: Occupational rheumatic diseases and upper limb strain in manual jobs in a light mechanical industry. Scand J Work Environ Health 5(Suppl 3):39–47, 1979.

Kurppa K, Waris P, Roklanen P: Tennis elbow: Lateral elbow pain syndrome. Scand J Work Environ Health 5(Suppl 3):15–18, 1979.

Luopajarvi T, Kuorinka I, Virolainen M, et al: Prevalence of tenosynovitis and other injuries of the upper extremities in repetitive work. Scand J Work Environ Health 5(Suppl 3):48–55, 1979.

Maeda K, Horiguchi S, Hosokawa M: History of the studies on occupational cervicobrachial disorder in Japan and remaining problems. J Hum Ergol 11:17–29, 1982.

Margolis W, Kraus JF: The prevalence of carpal tunnel syndrome symptoms in female supermarket checkers. J Occup Med 29:953–956, 1987.

Ranney DA, Wells RP, Moore A: Upper limb, musculoskeletal disorders in highly repetitive industries: Precise anatomical physical findings. Ergonomics 38:1408–1423, 1995.

Viikari-Juntura E: Neck and upper limb disorders among slaughterhouse workers: An epidemiologic study. Scand J Work Environ Health 9:283–290, 1983.

Viikari-Juntura E: Tenosynovitis, peritendinitis, and the tennis elbow syndrome. Scand J Work Environ Health *10*:443–449, 1984.

Wallace M, Buckle P: Ergonomic aspects of neck and upper limb disorders. Int Rev Ergonomics *1*:173–200, 1987.

Waris P: Occupational cervicobrachial syndromes: A review. Scand J Work Environ Heath *6*(Suppl 3):3–14, 1980.

3
Muscle Pathology With Overuse

Gisela Sjøgaard ———————————————————

Bente R. Jensen

Disorders of the locomotor system are found in a wide range of occupations and occur in connection with both heavy physical work and monotonous work. This is evident from a large number of epidemiologic studies (for references, see Chapter 2). However, such studies have not directly documented which specific form of exposure or work requirement is the cause of the disorder development. The mechanisms in the pathogenesis are an important element in this documentation. Different exposures have different effects on the tissues of the locomotor system in the form of morphologic or biochemical changes that can influence tissue function. Those factors that are shown to induce impaired function are regarded as potential risk factors. The presence of these factors during the performance of work implies a risk of disorder development, and prevention of such development can only be ensured by eliminating or minimizing the exposure to these risk factors and by ensuring adequate recovery following exposure.

The effect of such exposures may be an adaptation (a training effect) or an injury (a musculoskeletal disorder). The onset of injury is generally preceded by a long series of reactions in the tissues. Through knowledge of the various stages involved in such a developmental process, it is possible to initiate prevention before the injury arises, and before it becomes a chronic condition. This is in contrast to the information contributed by questionnaire-based epidemiologic studies, in which the actual development of musculoskeletal disorders among the employed is a necessary prerequisite for identification of potential risk factors. However, knowledge of the pathogenesis and of the importance of various physiologic states for development of musculoskeletal disorders is crucial for target-oriented prevention. Both pain and fatigue are essential phenomena in studies concerning mechanisms for development of disorders of the locomotor system.

PAIN

The perception of disorders of pain is naturally a subjective phenomenon. This perception does not reveal the cause of the pain. Depending on the location of the cause of the pain, a distinction is drawn between nociceptive, neurogenic, and psychogenic pain (Table 3–1), which are briefly discussed here (for more detail, see Chapter 6).

Nociceptive Pain

Pain that is triggered, for instance, from the skin, internal organs, tendons, or muscles (i.e., from the various peripheral tissues of the body) in conjunction with potentially tissue-damaging exposures is termed "nociceptive pain." For example, myogenic pain is nociceptive—pain that is triggered from the muscle itself. In many tissues, *special pain receptor organs* can be identified, but in the muscle-tendon complex, such organs have not been identified morphologically. However, there are many so-called *free nerve endings*, some of which specifically respond to noxious influences. They mediate the information to the central nervous system, from whence it is further mediated to the consciousness and triggers a perception of pain. These free nerve endings may be described as "functional pain receptors." Morphologically, the free nerve endings are situated in the interstitial space, that is, between the cells, such as between the muscle fibers. In the muscle-tendon complex, they are principally situated in the vicinity of muscle spindles, musculotendinous junctions, ten-

TABLE 3–1. Types of Pain According to Their Origin

TYPE	SOURCE OF PAIN
Nociceptive	Peripheral tissue (e.g., muscle)
Neurogenic	Direct irritation of nerve fiber (e.g., compression)
Psychogenic	Central nervous system (e.g., the brain)

don spindles, arterioles, venules, fat, and connective tissue (Stacey, 1969).

The free nerve endings respond to a large number of stimuli that may be both mechanical and chemical in character, some of which may be harmful to the tissue. Interstitial changes within the physiologic range of pH, inorganic phosphate, potassium, bradykinin, prostaglandin, arachidonic acid, serotonin, histamine, acetylcholine and the like will increase the firing frequency in the majority of free nerve endings that mediate pain perception (Johansson and Sojka, 1991; Mense, 1993; Mills et al., 1984). It should be observed that such chemical influences may be endogenic (i.e., produced as a result of physiologic processes in the tissue). More recent research shows that the free nerve endings may become sensitized, which means that exposure to a given chemical will now cause them to fire with higher frequency. Furthermore, the free nerve endings may develop a reduced threshold value for mechanical stimuli such as compressive, tensile, and shear forces. Finally, different simultaneous exposures may potentiate each other. For example, increased potassium concentration in the interstitium, as occurs in almost all muscular work, will increase sensitivity to the majority of other stimuli. Such modulations of the nerve response can play an important part in the development of allodynia, whereby stimuli that are not normally harmful to tissue will under such conditions convey a perception of pain (see Chapter 6).

Neurogenic Pain

Pain that is caused by *direct excitation of the sensory nerve fibers* and is not triggered via their relevant pain receptors or free nerve endings is termed "neurogenic pain." In our consciousness, we cannot distinguish where on the sensory nerve the action is taking place. The perception of pain is provided solely by the signals entering the central nervous system. This means that, irrespective of how the impulses in a nerve fiber are triggered, an increase of the impulse frequency in the nerve fiber is perceived as increasing pain from the area in which the nerve fiber's receptor organ (including free nerve endings) is situated. This is the explanation of so-called phantom pains, in which pain is experienced from, say, an amputated foot. In the same way, pain can be experienced in, for example, the hand or fingers as a result of proximal compression of the median nerve or other action directly on the nerve fiber. The same explanation is valid for the phenomenon known as "referred pain," which is used in diagnostics. Nociceptive (myogenic) and neurogenic pain together comprise the peripherally triggered pain forms, the cause of which lies outside the central nervous system.

Psychogenic Pain

Claims that musculoskeletal disorders are purely psychogenic— that is, that the cause of the pain is seated *entirely within the central nervous system*—are based on the fact that objective signs of actual damage to the peripheral tissue of the locomotor system are not always found in workers with work-related disorders. Psychogenically induced musculoskeletal disorders can naturally occur, but an assumption that this is the only possibility must be deemed erroneous or a radical simplification of the problem. For example, a number of studies have demonstrated an unusually high incidence of morphologic changes in persons with severe disorders (Henriksson, 1988; Larsson et al., 1988; Lindman et al., 1991). These studies are based on muscle biopsies, which naturally comprise very small tissue samples in order to avoid disabling the individuals concerned. Even a very local muscle injury triggers a general perception of pain from the whole of the muscle. If at this point in time a muscle biopsy is taken from the painful muscle, the likelihood of the sample containing any of the damaged tissue is very small, and the likelihood of a negative result is thus considerable. It must also be realized that injuries do not always manifest themselves as morphologic changes visible under the microscope. The interstitial space is very small (e.g., the distance between the muscle cells is only about 1 μm, or 10^{-6} m), and the identity of the substances that are able to trigger pain is largely still unknown. It is also uncertain whether chronic pain can occur after the original injury has healed, through the sensitization process described above. If tissue samples are taken during the chronic pain state, the cause of the pain may, for this reason, be unable to be documented as an abnormality in the samples.

Therefore, on the one hand, we must acknowledge that a considerable gulf exists in our knowledge of causal relationships between peripheral tissue changes and pain perception, and that there is a considerable need for both methodological and clinical research in this area. On the other hand, there exists today very extensive knowledge of morphologic and biochemical changes in muscles, nerves, and connective tissue (including tendons) resulting from different types of mechanical load. This is true both with regard to the manner in which function is influenced and with regard to which changes constitute risk factors for the tissue. The loads discussed in the present chapter are workloads that lead to physical/mechanical locomotor system exposures, and for which muscular effort must therefore be performed. Mental stresses can also lead to tissue exposures that constitute potential risk factors (Karasek and Theorell, 1990); these will be discussed in Chapter 17.

FATIGUE

When muscular work is performed over a prolonged period, fatigue develops. Fatigue may cause the work to be performed with less care or precision, whereby an accident can result. A fatigued worker is more likely to make a wrong movement, such as a slip and fall leading to injury. However, even if an accident does not occur, prolonged fatigue without adequate time for recovery can lead to the development of musculoskeletal disorders.

There are several definitions of muscle fatigue, one of which is the inability to sustain the expected or necessary development of external force or power. Use of this definition in a work physiology context would confine the term "muscle fatigue" to mean the point at which a specific job of work can no longer be performed with the same intensity. However, this point in time should more correctly be termed "exhaustion." The onset of the point of exhaustion is preceded by a large number of changes in the muscles that lead to diminished force-generating capacity. It is this phenomenon that is defined here as muscle fatigue, and that develops gradually from the beginning of every muscular effort.

A distinction is drawn between central and peripheral fatigue, depending on whether the fatigue arises proximally or distally to the motor end plate. Studies using external electrical stimulation of muscles show that muscle fatigue resulting from prolonged submaximal loads is principally of peripheral origin (Bigland-Ritchie et al., 1986; Merton et al., 1981). Thus, when fatigue arises in, for example, the shoulder muscles during prolonged working with the arms elevated (abducted/flexed), the physiologic causes of this fatigue must be sought locally in the shoulder region and not in the central nervous system.

Muscle contraction is a result of a long chain of interdependent processes. Muscle fatigue can theoretically be attributed to diminished function in each link of this chain. The significant physiologic factor for development of muscle fatigue may be mechanical, metabolic, or electrophysiologic in character. The last-mentioned can be recorded as changes in electromyographic (EMG) activity and used for objective documentation of work-related muscle fatigue. Depending on the physiologic load, the development of fatigue takes place quickly or slowly, and the point at which exhaustion occurs is dependent on the work intensity. This applies to both static and dynamic work (Fig. 3–1). For more basic information on muscle function, including the contractile process and muscle metabolism, the reader is referred to textbooks of muscle physiology (e.g., Jones and Round, 1990).

The processes that take place in conjunction with muscular effort are normally reversible. This means that muscles can recover when resting after exertion. A rest period following muscular activity is therefore essential to enable the muscle to recover its full functional capacity with regard to strength and endurance. There is no simple time equation for length of work and adequate length of subsequent resting period, because the process of physiologic recovery is dependent on the type of work that caused the muscle fatigue. If the fatigue is due to relatively high loads over a short period, the necessary recovery will be quicker than if the fatigue is due to prolonged working at low load levels. Thus, if the same muscle group or group of muscle fibers in a muscle are activated continuously for a full working day of 7or 8 hours, there is a risk that the muscle will not even be fully recovered by the next day.

The perception of fatigue is a very useful mechanism for protecting the muscles against overload. The work-induced increase in potassium concentration in the interstitial space possibly contributes to

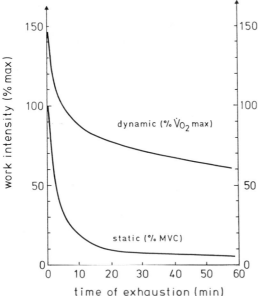

Figure 3–1. Muscular endurance increases with decreasing intensity of work. In the case of dynamic work, the intensity is stated as a percentage of the maximum oxygen uptake ($\dot{V}O_2$max). In the case of static contractions, the intensity is stated as a percentage of maximum voluntary contraction (MVC).

mediation of the perception of fatigue to the central nervous system (Sjøgaard, 1990). However, in situations of machine-controlled work or heavy work pressure, it is not always possible for an employee to take a rest when feeling fatigued. In other words, fatigue is ignored, which in the long term can have serious consequences.

Musculoskeletal disorders caused by physical/mechanical loads do not just occur in the workplace. For example, increasing attention is being given to the negative health effects of top-level sport, including the prevalence of sports injuries. Here also the cause is overloading, and sport is only good for the health when practiced in moderation. The nature of the work or sport determines which elements are the principal risk factors. In the working environment, there may be quite different physiologic mechanisms that cause diminished function in the case of heavy physical work compared with monotonous work. At worst, however, both strenuous work and monotony can inflict irreversible or chronic changes that may result in pain perception and impaired function.

CAUSAL MECHANISMS

Development of work-related pain and muscle fatigue is probably a result of a close interaction between mechanical and chemical factors. The body's physiologic reactions to muscular activity depend on the duration, frequency, and type of muscle contractions and the duration of the recovery. Depending on how these exposures are combined in the workplace, the effect of the work may be to improve physical working capacity or to overload and impair muscle function, as is seen in the work-related musculoskeletal disorders (Fig. 3–2).

Critical physiologic mechanisms are described here, with focus on (1) the motor control of movements, including the regulation of muscle force; (2) the mechanical forces and hydrostatic pressure generated in the tissues by muscle contractions and movements, and (3) the local circulatory and metabolic conditions.

Motor Control

Force regulation is performed by a muscle via "recruitment" (activation) of motor units. The motor unit is the smallest functional unit of a muscle and comprises a motor nerve together with the muscle fibers innervated by this nerve (i.e., activated by this motor nerve; see Fig. 3–3). The number of muscle fibers innervated by the same motor nerve range from a few to more than 1,000. The power of a

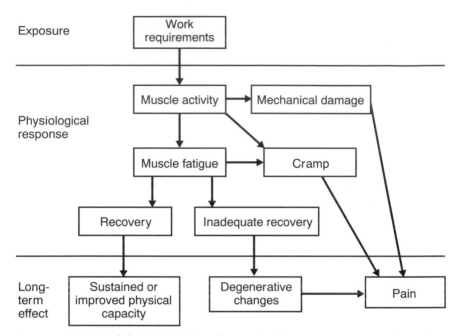

Figure 3–2. Model showing the relationship between exposure, physiological response, and long-term effects in the pathogenesis for development of work-related musculoskeletal disorders.

fresh muscle is regulated partly by the number of activated motor units and partly by modulation of the firing frequency of the active motor units (Fig. 3–4).

The recruitment pattern has major significance for the load on individual muscles. Even if the muscle as a whole is working to only a relatively small part of its capacity, and therefore generating a small percentage of its maximum voluntary contraction (MVC) force, as, for example, during monotonous work, individual motor units (and thus also their muscle cells) may very well be working at high or even very high relative load. This is because only a small number of that muscle's motor units are activated at low loads. Work-related disorders are a frequent occurrence with monotonous work; symptoms may develop just because only a relatively few motor units in the muscle are recruited and the load is not distributed equally among all fibers of the muscle.

The recruitment of motor units often takes place according to a hierarchical pattern in which units with a low threshold value are activated at low force levels, whereas others are only recruited at high force levels (Fig. 3–5). Each time a motor unit is activated, it generates approximately 30 per cent of MVC. This means that, even if a specific job demands a mean load of only 10 per cent of MVC, the relatively

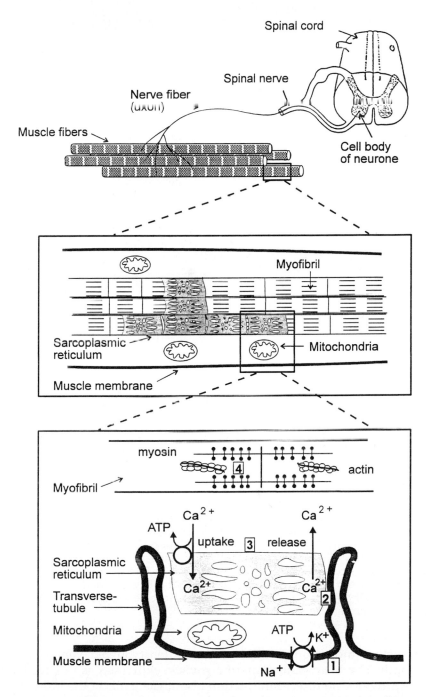

Figure 3–3. Diagrammatic representation of a motor unit in combination with an enlargement of a muscle fiber and a further enlargement of subcellular structures of a muscle fiber. In the latter part of the figure are indicated (*1*) action potential propagation along muscle membrane and T tubuli; (*2*) coupling of T-tubular charge movement with sarcoplasmic reticulum (SR) Ca^{2+} release; (*3*) SR Ca^{2+} release and reuptake; and (*4*) actin-myosin ATP reaction and crossbridge cycling.

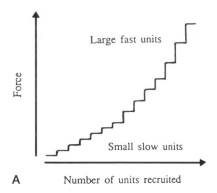

A   Number of units recruited

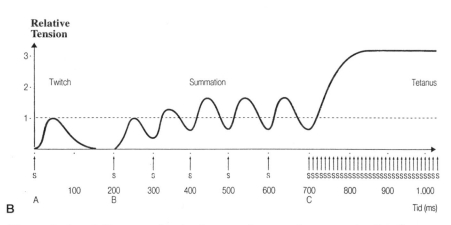

B

Figure 3–4. *A,* Force graduation by recruitment of motor units. Small motor units are recruited first; with increasing force, larger motor units are recruited having higher threshold levels. *B,* Force graduation by frequency modulation of a motor unit. Twitch force is about one third of tetanic force and, with summation force, can be gradually increased to tetanic force. (Adapted by permission from Jones DA, Round JM: Skeletal Muscle in Health and Disease: A Textbook of Muscle Pathology. Manchester, England, Manchester University Press, 1990.)

few active motor units will muster at least 30 per cent of their strength. The force generation of a muscle expressed as relative load thus provides no direct information about the load on the individual motor unit.

Several studies indicate that, in monotonous work, it is the same motor units with low threshold value that are active continuously (i.e., work from early until late); these may be termed "Cinderella fibers" (Hägg, 1991; Sejersted and Vøllestad, 1993). If the same work

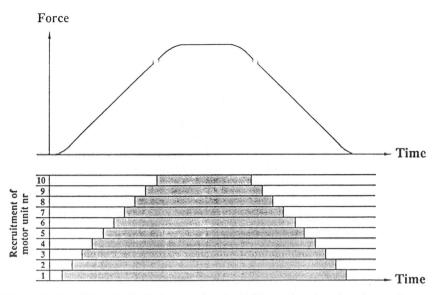

Figure 3–5. Schematic diagram showing a hierarchical-ordered recruitment of the motor units. *Top curve*: Force development. *Bottom curve*: Recruitment. (Adapted with permission from Hägg GM: Static work load and occupational myalgia. A new explanation model. *In* Anderson PA, Hobart DJ, Danoff, JA (eds): Electromyographical Kinesiology. Amsterdam, Elsevier Science Publishers BV, 1991, pp 141–144.)

is performed day after day, this stereotyped recruitment pattern will lead to fatigue and possible overload of these continuously activated fibers. Some studies of muscle biopsies from persons with work-related musculoskeletal disorders have demonstrated changes in individual muscle cells, such as irregular fibers, moth-eaten fibers, and ragged red fibers, of which the last type belongs to motor units with low threshold value (Henriksson, 1988; Larsson et al., 1988; Lindman et al., 1991). One well-supported hypothesis points to the likelihood that local metabolic changes resulting from a stereotypical recruitment pattern can lead to a reflex propagation, via the gamma system, to further activate muscle fibers (Johansson and Sojka, 1991). This may induce a self-perpetuating vicious circle as more and more fibers are activated reflexly, fatigued, and overloaded, with a consequent perception of pain.

Mechanical Forces

The forces that are generated in muscles, tendons, and connective tissue are dependent on active muscle force development, both at the muscle level and at the individual motor unit level. To this must be added the external forces that affect the locomotor system.

The different types of mechanical forces that occur in muscles, tendons, and connective tissue include tensile forces, shear forces, and frictional forces. The magnitude of the tensile forces and shear forces in both cases is principally related to (1) the magnitude of force development, (2) the recruitment pattern, and (3) the architecture of the muscles. The frictional forces arise from movement of different tissues relative to each other. The actual exposure as a result of the mechanical forces will also depend on whether the muscle is in a fresh or fatigued state and whether edema is present in the tissue.

When the internal forces exceed the point of failure for the tissue, acute injury occurs. This may be in the form of a bone fracture, prolapsed disk, ruptured tendon, or torn muscle fibers. It commonly occurs with heavy physical work. A clear distinction must be made between damage to the locomotor system caused by acute injuries (which should be reported and recorded as accidents), and damage arising from prolonged overload (which can result in musculoskeletal disorders and should be reported as such).

The forces that occur in the muscles depend both on the activation level and on the type of contraction (e.g., static versus dynamic, or concentric versus eccentric[1]). The muscles are capable of mustering their greatest forces during eccentric contractions (i.e., when exerting a braking effort). If the force development is relatively high, although not high enough to exceed the point of failure of the tissue, microruptures can occur, particularly during eccentric effort. If such microruptures are inflicted repeatedly without sufficient time for recovery, the regenerative processes become inadequate. This can lead to degenerative and inflammatory processes in tendons, muscles, discs, and joints. Depending on the tissue, different types of microruptures or microtraumas occur. In muscles, for example, ruptures of myofibrils (Z-band streaming) have been observed (Fridén, 1984). Exposure to high forces may also be reflected in the formation of intracellular vacuoles, swollen mitochondria, and increased intracellular water. Such changes are seen in conjunction with muscle soreness and pain after unaccustomed heavy work or after excessively hard training in sport activities.

However, these intracellular changes cannot be registered by the sensory nerves, since their free endings are located extracellulary in

---

[1]During static contractions, the muscle fibers remain at the same length during tension development, whereas during dynamic contractions, they change length, performing concentric work during shortening and eccentric work during lengthening.

the interstitial space. Only if the muscle cell membrane develops a leak, so that changes take place in the chemical composition of the interstitial phase, can a perception of pain result. The actual occurrence of such an event is documented by increased blood concentration of, for example, the muscle enzymes creatine kinase and myoglobin (Newham et al., 1986). Extracellular changes further occur as a result of ruptures in elastin and collagen, whereby the extracellular matrix structure of proteoglycans is changed (Stauber et al., 1990). Finally, effusions of blood from damaged blood vessels will lead to liberation of bradykinin from plasma proteins, which is capable of sensitizing the free nerve endings (Mense, 1993).

More recent studies show that repeated eccentric contractions, even at relatively low contraction levels, can diminish muscle function. For example, 20 minutes of eccentric contractions at 15 per cent of MVC performed at 3-second intervals was found to produce increased intramuscular resting pressure, muscle edema, increased muscle fiber area, Z-band streaming, and muscle enzymes in the blood. The subjective signs of muscle injuries were muscle soreness and stiffness, principally 1 to 2 days after the work. The same protocol performed with concentric contractions failed to show corresponding muscle changes (Hargens et al, 1989). When evaluating the load during highly repetitive work, it is therefore vitally important to consider the type of muscle contraction.

In the case of selective recruitment of individual motor units in monotonous work, the muscle tension will be distributed to a relatively small number of the muscle fibers. The magnitude of the forces in the muscles will therefore be dependent on the longitudinal change in the individual muscle fibers during contraction. This can probably explain the mechanical microruptures that are found at even relatively low load levels. The microruptures probably occur in the endomysium (the connective tissue surrounding each individual muscle fiber) as well as in the individual muscle cells.

During muscle contractions, the relative movement between the soft tissues of the body, and between these tissues and bones, causes friction between the tissues. At some places in the body, this friction, if repeated frequently, may result in tissue irritation and overloading. This mechanical component is relevant, among others, in the development of carpal tunnel syndrome, which is discussed further in Chapter 11. Besides producing pain, this form of mechanical tissue irritation can also cause degenerative changes to the tissues (Armstrong et al., 1984).

If the processes that trigger pain lead the worker to reduce the muscle force, then regenerative processes may become dominant and tissue recovery begins. If sufficient recovery is permitted, the result may be stronger tissue—that is, a training effect has occurred.

Intramuscular Pressure

When a muscle contracts, the hydrostatic pressure in the muscle increases. In certain muscles, the intramuscular pressure rises to 400 to 500 mm Hg at maximum force development. The maximum intramuscular pressure that develops in a fresh muscle during a muscle contraction varies considerably from muscle to muscle and depends primarily on the anatomy of the muscle and its surroundings, such as whether the muscle is thin or bulky and whether its location is deep or superficial (Järvholm, 1990; Jensen et al., 1995a; Sejersted and Hargens, 1986). For example, the intramuscular pressure in the infraspinatus muscle, and particularly in the supraspinatus, is four to five times as high as in the deltoideus or trapezius at the same relative load (Fig. 3–6).

Muscle activity leads to an increase in muscle water content. At high dynamic work intensities, the muscle volume may increase by 10 to 20 per cent in the course of a few minutes (Sjøgaard, 1990). However, fluid is also accumulated in the muscles during prolonged static muscle contractions at 5 to 10 per cent of MVC; in other words, the muscles become edematous. Fluid accumulation leads to thickening of the muscle. If the arms are held abducted at an angle of 30 degrees, the thickness of the supraspinatus muscle increases after just 10 minutes, and will be increased by approximately 15 per cent after 30 minutes (Jensen et al., 1994). For muscles situated in delimited, closed muscle compartments with low compliance in, for example, the shoulder region (supraspinatus and infraspinatus) or leg (tibialis anterior), an increase in fluid content can lead to increased intramuscular pressure with consequent risk of development of a compartment syndrome. This condition is well known in the muscle compartments of the leg (Pedowitz et al., 1990; Styf and Körner, 1987). Edema arising in one muscle compartment does not spread to the adjacent compartments, which prolongs the time before fluid balance is returned to normal.

The fluid balance in the muscles is regulated by the net fluid displacement across the capillaries, the transport of fluid to the lymphatic system, and the capacity of the lymphatic system. Each of these three factors represents a dynamically complex system that is influenced during muscle contractions. At high work intensities, the osmotic gradient plays an important role, whereas, during prolonged, static muscular effort, a significant cause for the muscle edema is the filtration of fluid out of the capillaries, together with impaired fluid transport to the lymphatic system and reduced lymphatic system capacity.

When the intramuscular pressure rises during a muscle contraction, the local blood supply is affected, even at contractions of just a few

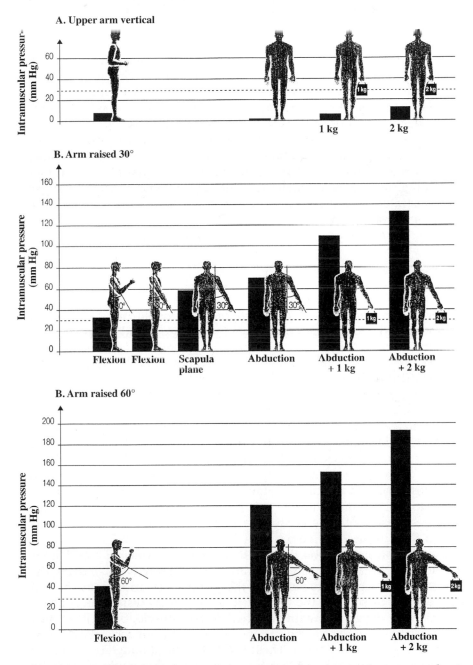

Figure 3–6. Intramuscular pressure measured in supraspinatus muscle at different arm positions. *A*, Upper arm vertical. *B*, Arm elevated 30 degrees, and arm elevated 60 degrees.

per cent of MVC. Muscle function is dependent on an adequate blood supply, by which substrate is delivered to and metabolites are removed from the muscles. As a result of the substantial differences in intramuscular pressure from muscle to muscle at the same relative load, both the circulatory and metabolic conditions are also very different. Insufficient blood supply and changes in the chemical balance of muscles are significant causes of muscle inability to withstand prolonged increases in intramuscular pressure. Studies in which intramuscular pressure is increased by external compression for periods corresponding to a working day have shown that pressures of approximately 30 mm Hg and above, maintained for a prolonged time, lead to muscle damage that can be objectively quantified 48 hours following the pressure increase. The physiologic muscle changes demonstrated by muscle pressures of this magnitude and above are histologic changes in the form of fiber atrophy, fiber splitting, edema, and decreased muscle oxygen tension (Hargens et al., 1981).

Blood Flow

Tissue function depends on an adequate blood supply. However, it is not always clear what constitutes "adequate blood supply" for a specific work. A large number of physiologic regulatory mechanisms constantly endeavor to optimize the blood flow, but the capacity may be insufficient, which can lead to a muscle energy crisis.

During prolonged static muscle contractions, blood flow to the active muscles is increased (e.g., as a result of increased blood pressure). The increase in blood pressure is dependent on the relative muscle load. In addition, however, static contractions involving large muscle groups (e.g., the back muscles) trigger a greater blood pressure response than do those involving small muscle groups (e.g., the arm muscles). Thus, in the case of monotonous work involving prolonged static loading of small muscle groups, this means that the blood pressure response will only contribute to a rather small increase in the blood flow in these active muscles.

Cardiac output can be the limiting factor for muscle blood flow, particularly during intensive, dynamic whole-body work. During the muscle contractions themselves, the local circulation may be occluded, but as soon as the muscle relaxes, a reperfusion takes place. In this way oxygen is again supplied to the muscle, but at the same time relatively high concentrations of free oxygen radicals may be formed (Sjödin et al., 1990). These are toxic and damage biologic cell membranes by breaking down the membrane phospholipids (Lovlin et al., 1987). Frequently repeated relatively forceful muscle contractions (highly repetitive, high-force work) may in this way cause accumulation of free radicals, resulting in a cell-damaging process at the membrane level.

The degree of vascularization (capillary density) in the individual tissues, and the location of the peripheral vessels relative to bones, for instance, are also of great importance for the local blood supply during static muscle contractions. The vascular supply and the nerve supply to the cranial part of the infraspinatus muscle as well as to the supraspinatus tendon all run through the supraspinatus muscle compartment. This means that a prolonged increased muscle pressure in this muscle compartment will also have significance both for the blood supply and nerve function to the infraspinatus and for the blood supply to the relatively poorly vascularized insertion of the supraspinatus on the head of the humerus.

During static contractions, the blood flow through the smallest blood vessels, the capillaries, is especially diminished by the increased intramuscular pressure. Studies of intramuscular pressures and regulation of blood flow at static loads, combined with microvascular studies of blood flow, have led to a hypothesis that explains a possible link between prolonged monotonous work and the development of muscle pain. Some of the white blood cells (granulocytes) can, under certain physical conditions, reduce the microcirculation by blocking a significant number of the capillaries in a purely mechanical way. This process is known as "granulocyte plugging." Granulocytes are not normally present at the capillary level but rather are shunted past. However, when the smooth musculature of the blood vessels is relaxed (vasodilation), the granulocytes may flow into the capillaries. If, at the same time, the pressure difference between the arterial and venous ends of the capillary is very small, the granulocytes will not be able to pass through. Precisely these two conditions are present during low static loads as they occur in monotonous work in muscles that typically are prone to the development of work-related musculoskeletal disorders. This is because (1) metabolite accumulation triggers vasodilation and (2) a low increase in blood pressure and an increased tissue pressure combine to reduce the driving pressure (i.e., the pressure gradient from the arterial to the venous end of the capillaries (Jensen et al., 1995b).

The phenomenon of granulocyte plugging is known from ischemic cardiac diseases and from situations in which individuals have suffered from heavy blood loss (Schmid-Schönbein and Engler, 1988). The granulocytes leave the microvascular network for the extracellular space amid formation of free radicals and an increase in capillary wall permeability. The free radicals are toxic and especially harmful to the biologic cell membranes, and arachidonic acid and prostaglandins may be formed at the same time. As previously described, these two substances can stimulate nociceptors and cause a pain sensation from the muscle. This hypothesis may thus explain a possible link between pain perception and morphologic and biochemical changes that may result from prolonged monotonous work.

Metabolic Factors

When muscles actively contract and develop force, they convert chemically bound energy into mechanical energy. However, the store of chemically bound energy in the muscles is limited (Vøllestad and Sejersted, 1988). This applies, for example, to the store of carbohydrates in the form of glycogen. It is therefore important that the muscle can be continuously provided with adequate supplies of new substrates, including oxygen, during the work. This is necessary for the formation of adenosine triphosphate (ATP), and only ATP-bound energy can be converted into mechanical energy in the myofibrils. If no ATP is present, muscle cramp—which is extremely painful—will develop (Fig. 3–2). The mechanisms of this pain development are largely unknown and may be fundamentally different from work-related muscle pain. Voluntary muscle contractions do not appear capable of reducing ATP concentration by more than 20 to 30 per cent. It is conceivable that the development of fatigue is a protective mechanism that ensures that ATP depletion, with attendant cramps and irreversible reactions in the muscle tissue, cannot normally take place.

Many studies have shown a close relationship between fatigue or exhaustion and depletion of glycogen in individual muscle fibers. Disagreement exists on whether reduced glycogen concentration in muscles is a direct cause of fatigue, but there is no sign that it may be a risk factor for development of muscle pain. Indirectly, however, depletion of glycogen from certain muscle fibers can mean that other fibers must work harder and may thus become overloaded.

Accumulation of metabolites, such as lactic acid, takes place during intensive work and is accompanied by a fall in tissue pH (i.e., increase in hydrogen ion [H^+] concentration). Thereby, a key enzyme is inhibited in the process of glycolysis that might play a role in fatigue development. It is more likely, however, that it is the increase in H^+ concentration itself that has an inhibiting effect on the contractile filaments, including a reduction in the sensitivity of troponin to calcium ion Ca^{2+}. Low pH values can also stimulate the free nerve endings and thus trigger a pain perception. However, it is not likely that lactate accumulation within physiologic levels has a damaging effect on tissue. Moreover, pain and morphologic changes can very well arise in situations in which lactate and pH are at resting level.

Changes in the electrolyte balance affect muscle function. All forms of muscular effort are accompanied by a continuous loss of potassium ion (K^+) from the intracellular space of the muscle fibers. This can play an important part in the development of fatigue because the K^+ gradient across the cell membrane is crucial for activation of the muscle fiber via the motor nerve. The duration of the subsequent recovery can also depend on, among other things, the magnitude of K^+ loss. This fatigue mechanism, although possibly a useful protective device, may be ignored, particularly at prolonged low levels of contraction (Sjøgaard, 1990). As with H^+, an increased K^+ concentration in the interstitial space can mediate a perception of pain by sensitizing free nerve endings. It is not likely that changes in K^+ have a harmful effect on tissue directly. However, increased extracellular K^+ may lead to a flux of Ca^{2+} from the extracellular to the intracellular space in the muscle fibers, and this can have a damaging effect on the muscle fibers.

During muscle activity, the actin-myosin reaction is initiated in the myofibrils through liberation of Ca^{2+} from the sarcoplasmic reticulum to the cytosol, as shown in Figure 3–3. The return transport of Ca^{2+} from cytosol to sarcoplasmic reticulum also requires ATP, and, when the formation of ATP is inadequate, a buildup of Ca^{2+} in the cytosol may result. To this must be added the previously mentioned possibility of a flux of Ca^{2+} from the extracellular to the intracellular space. In conclusion, therefore, prolonged heavy work means that the concentration of free Ca^{2+} in the cytosol will be increased for a prolonged period. A possible contributory factor is that the sensitivity to Ca^{2+} in the contractile filaments may be reduced and that an increased Ca^{2+} concentration is now necessary for initiation of the contraction process. The pathogenesis of Ca^{2+}-induced muscular degeneration has been studied very closely, and it has been shown that Ca^{2+} stimulates the phospholipase and also increases the sensitivity of the membrane lipids to free radicals. Both of these mechanisms lead to a breakdown of the muscle cell membrane. In addition, the increased Ca^{2+} concentration induces a Ca^{2+} overload of the mitochondria in which the Ca^{2+} accumulates and the formation of ATP is inhibited (Fig. 3–7). In this way, working capacity is reduced and a vicious circle is created (Edwards, 1988). Factors contributing to work-related pain and fatigue are summarized in Table 3–2.

OPTIMIZATION OF WORKLOAD

As mentioned at the beginning of this chapter, the effect on the locomotor system of a physical/mechanical exposure may be either

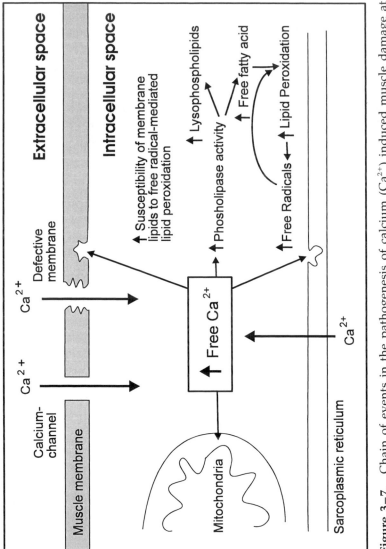

Figure 3–7. Chain of events in the pathogenesis of calcium (Ca^{2+}) induced muscle damage at the cell level (a further enlargement of the lower part in Fig. 3–3). Such mechanisms may play a role in the development of work-related disorders and injuries.

TABLE 3–2. Possible Mechanisms Involved in Development of
Work-Related Fatigue and Pain

Motor Control
Task related recruitment pattern induces high relative load on a few
("Cinderella") muscle fibers

Mechanical Forces (tensile, shear, friction)
Myofibrillar rupture, release of chemicals inducing inflammatory response

Intramuscular Pressure
Increase with muscle tension, as well as contraction-induced fluid shifts,
interfering with blood flow by reducing driving pressure and increasing
local resistance

Muscle Blood Flow
Insufficient driving pressure through capillaries impairs blood flow in spite
of metabolic vasodilation
Granulocyte plugging, free radical formation

Metabolic Crises
Drop in pH and increased extracellular $[K^+]$ may trigger pain perception
Prolonged increased intracellular $[Ca^{2+}]$ may damage muscle

positive, in the form of training, or negative, in the form of injury or
disorder. In the workplace health and safety field, considerable attention has been focused on prevention of work-related musculoskeletal
disorders by minimizing the physical load on the body. However, as
muscle training physiology has clearly shown, a well-functioning
body is dependent on a certain amount of physical activity. With
inactivity, the degenerative processes will assume command and the
various tissues of the locomotor system will atrophy (Fig. 3–8).

Increased attention should therefore be given to optimizing, rather
than minimizing, the physical activity of the individual at work.
Where work is optimized in accordance with ergonomic principles,
it is possible to maintain muscle function, and possibly even create a
muscle training effect for the individual person.

Work optimization means

• Reducing local mechanical loads that exceed the tissue point
of failure.
• Reducing work intensity so that it does not exceed the body's
energy metabolism capacity.
• Avoiding prolonged static muscular loads.
• Avoiding prolonged highly repetitive work.
• Ensuring adequate recovery after each work period.

In many jobs, the workload is traditionally determined by the function and design of the production system. However, the knowledge

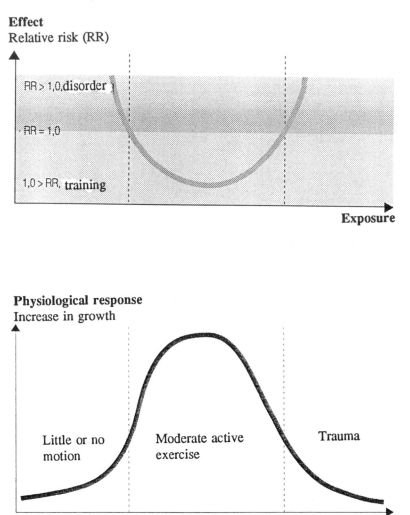

Figure 3–8. There is no simple correlation between the magnitude of the exposure and the physiologic response of the body. In order to avoid negative effects on the body, the exposure should be optimized. There is a certain mechanical load at which maximum tissue growth and maintenance of function are achieved. Similarly, there is a certain degree of exposure at which there is minimum risk of attrition. At best, a training effect may even be achieved.

of work physiology and ergonomics should be incorporated into the design phase of new production systems. The close relationship between production systems and human workload renders a change of workload difficult in established production processes. Accordingly, adverse workplaces will continue to exist for many years. In those cases in which it is considered harmful to health to perform a given work process for the whole working day, day after day, it may be necessary to limit the amount of time each individual employee spends on that process. The rest of the time must be devoted to other tasks, thus providing each individual with a varied job profile. This is beneficial not only from the viewpoint of the physical-mechanical loads, but also with regard to the psychological load, as discussed in Chapter 17. Preventative efforts in the future must, among other things, concentrate on job design based on these principles.

REFERENCES

Armstrong TJ, Castelli WA, Evans FG, et al: Some histological changes in carpal tunnel contents and their biomechanical implications. J Occup Med 26:197–201, 1984.

Bigland-Ritchie B, Furbush F, Woods J: Fatigue of intermittent submaximal voluntary contractions: Central and peripheral factors. J Appl Physiol 61: 421–429, 1986.

Edwards RHT: Hypotheses of peripheral and central mechanisms underlying occupational muscle pain and injury. Eur J Appl Physiol 57:275–281, 1988.

Fridén J: Muscle soreness after exercise: Implications of morphological changes. Int J Sports Med 5:57–66, 1984.

Hägg GM: Static work loads and occupational myalgia: A new explanation model. In Anderson PA, Hobart DJ, Danoff JV (eds): Electromyographical Kinesiology. Amsterdam, Elsevier Science Publishers BV, 1991, pp 141–144.

Hägg GM: Zero crossing rate as an index of electromyographic spectral alterations and its applications to ergonomics. Arbete och Hälsa 5:1–37, 1991.

Hargens AR, Parazynski S, Aratow M, et al: Muscle changes with eccentric exercise: Implications on earth and in space. In Benzi G (ed): Advances in Myochemistry. London, John Libbey Eurotext Ltd, 1989, pp 299–312.

Hargens AR, Schmidt DA, Evans KL, et al: Quantitation of skeletal-muscle necrosis in a model compartment syndrome. J Bone Joint Surg 63A:631–636, 1981.

Henriksson KG: Muscle pain in neuromuscular disorders and primary fibromyalgia. Eur J Appl Physiol 57:348–352, 1988.

Järvholm U: On shoulder muscle load: An experimental study of muscle pressures, EMG and blood flow. Doctoral thesis, University of Göteborg Press, 1990.

Jensen BR, Jørgensen K, Huijing PA, et al: Soft tissue architecture and intramuscular pressure in the shoulder region. Eur J Morphol 3:205–220, 1995a.

Jensen BR, Jørgensen K, Sjøgaard G: The effect of prolonged isometric contractions on muscle fluid balance. Eur J Appl Physiol 69:439–444, 1994.

Jensen BR, Sjøgaard G, Bornmyr S, et al: Intramuscular laser-Doppler flowmetry in the supraspinatus muscle during isometric contractions. Eur J Appl Physiol 72:373–378, 1995b.

Johansson H, Sojka P: Pathophysiological mechanisms involved in genesis and spread of muscular tension in occupational muscle pain and in chronic musculoskeletal pain syndromes: A hypothesis. Med Hypotheses 35:196–203, 1991.

Jones DA, Round JM: Skeletal Muscle in Health and Disease: A Textbook of Muscle Physiology. Manchester, England, Manchester University Press, 1990.

Karasek R, Theorell T: Healthy Work: Stress, Productivity and the Reconstruction of Working Life. New York, Basic Books, 1990.

Larsson SE, Bengtsson A, Bodegård L, et al: Muscle changes in work-related chronic myalgia. Acta Orthop Scand 59:552–556, 1988.

Lindman R, Hagberg M, Änqvist KA, et al: Changes in muscle morphology in chronic trapezius myalgia. Scand J Work Environ Health 17:347–355, 1991.

Lovlin R, Cottle W, Pyke I, et al: Are indices of free radical damage related to exercise intensity? Eur J Appl Physiol 56:313–316, 1987.

Mense S: Nociception from skeletal muscle in relation to clinical muscle pain: Review article. Pain 54:241–289, 1993.

Merton PA, Hill DK, Morton HB: Indirect and direct stimulation of fatigued human muscle. Ciba Found Symp 82:120–129, 1981.

Mills KR, Newham DJ, Edward RHT: Muscle pain. In Wall PO, Melzack R (eds): Textbook of Pain. New York, Churchill Livingstone, 1984, pp 319–330.

Newham DJ, Jones DA, Edwards RHT: Plasma creatine kinase changes after eccentric and concentric contractions. Muscle Nerve 9:59–63, 1986.

Pedowitz RA, Hargens AR, Mubarak SJ, et al: Modified criteria for the objective diagnosis of chronic compartment syndrome of the leg. Am J Sports Med 18:35–40, 1990.

Schmid-Schonbein GW, Engler RL: Granulocyte capillary plugging in myocardial ischemia. In Manabe M, Zweifach BW, Messmer K (eds): Microcirculation in Circulatory Disorders. Tokyo, Springer-Verlag, 1988, pp 327–335.

Sejersted OM, Hargens AR: Regional pressure and nutrition of skeletal muscle during isometric contraction. In Hargens AR (ed): Tissue Nutrition and Viability. New York, Springer-Verlag, 1986, pp 263–284.

Sejersted OM, Vøllestad NK: Physiology of muscle fatigue and associated pain. In Værøy H, Merskey H (eds): Progress in Fibromyalgia and Myofascial Pain. Amsterdam, Elsevier Science Publishers BV, 1993, pp 41–51.

Sjodin B, Hellsten Westling Y, Apple FS: Biochemical mechanisms for oxygen free radical formation during exercise. Sports Med 10:236–254, 1990.

Sjøgaard G: Exercise-induced muscle fatigue: The significance of potassium. Acta Physiol Scand 140(Suppl 593):1–64, 1990.

Stacey MJ: Free nerve endings in skeletal muscle of the cat. J Anat 105:231–254, 1969.

Stauber WT, Clarkson PM, Fritz VK, et al: Extracellular matrix disruption and pain after eccentric muscle action. J Appl Physiol 69:868–874, 1990.

Styf JR, Körner LM: Diagnosis of chronic anterior compartment syndrome in the lower leg. Acta Orthop Scand 58:139–144, 1987.

Vøllestad NK, Sejersted OM: Biochemical correlates of fatigue: A brief review. Eur J Appl Physiol 57:336–347, 1988.

4
Task Analysis

Richard Wells

It is noted in Chapter 8 that a diagnosis of work-related musculo-skeletal injuries should be based on a *specific pathologic change* to an *identified tissue* subjected to *sufficient stress at work* to produce *characteristic symptoms* verified by *specific tests*. In epidemiologic literature, the term "work-related musculoskeletal disorders" (WMSDs) is used to include these as well as less precisely diagnosed problems that appear to be related to physical stress at work. The purpose of this chapter is to outline methods for the determination of *stress at work*—that is, the tissue loads that might induce potential pathologic change in tissue during work. The same information can also be used to determine whether the work will be likely to load specific tissues that have already been injured. This process is called task analysis.

The information derived from a task analysis has potential use

1. In reducing the stressors acting on the musculoskeletal system and thereby reducing the number of workers that might develop WMSDs (primary prevention).

2. In aiding those already injured to return to work with reduced risk of recurrence (secondary prevention). This is accomplished by identification of tasks or elements of tasks that may aggravate or reinjure previously injured tissue.

The work and the worker's ability to perform it can be studied in many ways. This chapter primarily deals with task analysis, but it also addresses topics important in the complex issue of *job matching*.

This usually entails a comparison of a *physical demands analysis* with a *functional capacity assessment* (also known as a functional abilities evaluation) of an individual, which reveals which aspects of the job the individual cannot perform. The importance of job matching is briefly discussed in Chapter 14. Physical demands analysis involves an extended job description, including physical requirements such as bending, kneeling, or lifting, which are part of the scope of this chapter, as well as requirements for vision and hearing. For more information, the interested reader is referred to texts such as *Fitness for Work* (Frazer, 1992).

As part of a job-matching process, changes are often suggested in the job that would enable a particular individual to be accommodated. These changes will often make the job easier and less potentially injurious to able-bodied workers as well.

RISK FACTORS FOR MUSCULOSKELETAL DISORDERS

Chapter 5 will review musculoskeletal disorders and conclude that many musculoskeletal disorders exhibit associations with work. For some tissues and disorders, there is evidence that work exposures are associated with the development of injury and that the relative risk of certain work exposures is high. This has been shown to be true for shoulder and hand/wrist tendinitis, low back pain, carpal tunnel syndrome, hypothenar hammer syndrome, and tension neck syndrome. Plausible biologic mechanisms by which these risk factors result in disorders of the musculoskeletal system have been proposed but, strictly speaking, evidence of causation has not been shown experimentally. Despite this, our best evidence points to a complex interaction of physical (ergonomic), psychosocial, and individual factors in the production of musculoskeletal disorders at work.

The studies referred to above also uncovered specific attributes of work that were related to the development of WMSDs (Table 4–1). These included non-neutral postures, forceful exertions, constrained or static postures, repetitive work, use of pinch grip, work over shoulder height, prolonged periods of time with the trunk inclined forward, heavy lifting, twisting while lifting, and both whole-body and segmentally applied vibration. These are termed risk factors for the development of WMSD. It is difficult to imagine any work without some of these risk factors present, and one can quickly fall into the mindset that work is inherently dangerous and the observation of a bent wrist during work implies hazard.

TABLE 4-1. Unfavorable Working Conditions and Their
Potential Effects*

Risk Factors Present at Work	Possible Tissue Changes	Example Diagnoses
High forces/ moments	Strain in tendons or muscles; high forces for short duration may lead to tissue disruption; moderate forces for long durations may lead to creep in tendons or muscle fatigue	Tendinitis Muscle strain
Exertion of force in nonoptimal postures	Increased fatigue	Muscle pain, forearm myalgia
Extreme posture	Compression of blood vessels or nerves	Carpal tunnel syndrome
Overhead work	Increased intramuscular pressure in supraspinatus with reduction in blood flow	Myalgia of the trapezius and/or supraspinatus and supraspinatus tendinitis
Whole body vibration	Increased shrinkage of intervertebral discs	Low pack pain
Hand/arm vibration	Increased grip force to maintain control of object Damage to nervous tissue	Increased fatigue and muscle pain Carpal tunnel syndrome Raynaud's disease
Immobile posture	Static contraction of muscles	Myalgia/tension neck syndrome
High-frequency movements	High velocity of tendon sliding combined with static contraction of more proximal muscles	Tenosynovitis Myalgia/tension neck syndrome

*These health effects are based on epidemiologic studies, and the presence of the risk factor increases the risk of an individual developing WMSD. All potential health effects depend on the length of exposure to the conditions, the magnitude or size of the stressor, and the variation of the exposure.

A distinction is made in industrial hygiene between toxicity and hazard. Benzene is highly toxic, yet, if used infrequently and in small concentrations (a person's exposure is low), the hazard is small. Similarly, even for wrist flexion close to an individual's range of motion, the risk is also low if the motion is infrequent. In fact, the adoption of "extreme postures" for short periods of time is beneficial; they are called stretch breaks. In general, assessment of the load on tissues of the musculoskeletal system requires consideration of not only the size of the load but also its variation through time. An infrequent high load or a continuous low load may both cause problems for workers.

In general work is positive, both physically and mentally, and the purpose of task analysis for use in the prevention and treatment of WMSD is to describe the elements of the job and then identify the potentially adverse aspects of work (risk factors) so that they may be eliminated or the hazard associated with them reduced.

Assessment of moment of force, posture, static exertion, frequency, and psychosocial factors allows insight into the injury potential of work tasks. Studies of the work relatedness of jobs have identified three major classes or risk factors: (1) the forces exerted in the job, (2) the postures of the arms and trunk, and (3) the time elements of the job (frequency or duration of activities). This section introduces a number of key concepts that relate the notions of force, posture, and time to the jobs people do and that are useful in helping clinicians and others observe and describe work.

Joint Moment of Force

The joint moment of force expresses the commonplace notion that the turning effect (or tendency to cause rotation) of a load about a pivot point depends both on the size of the load and on the distance of the load from the pivot. The joint moment of force (also known as the joint moment or joint torque) accounts for both these facts by multiplying the force by the distance (Fig. 4–1). If the load is known in Newtons and the distance in meters, the moment is in Newton-meters, or N·m (in the imperial system, the force may be in pounds and the distance in feet, giving a moment in ft-lb).

This simple concept can be used to estimate the loading on, for example, the tissues of the shoulder and low back. The joint moment of force caused by external loads must be resisted internally by the muscles and ligaments surrounding the joint; the higher the moment, the higher the loads on the tissues of that joint (Fig. 4–2). The joint moment of force, or torque, can be one of the best predictors of the injury potential of a task (Marras et al., 1993). In addition, there are estimates of average strengths at many joints, also expressed in terms of joint moment. A comparison of task requirements with these maximum capacities can give a relative measure of task demand.

The joint moment of force can be used to explain how people can lift heavy weights under some circumstances, yet even light loads, under adverse conditions, can create potentially injurious loading on the body. Figure 4–2 shows the loading on the back, in terms of joint moment, when lifting a 10-kg (~20-lb) load in two different positions,

Moment = Load X Distance

Balanced: L1 x D1 = L2 x D2

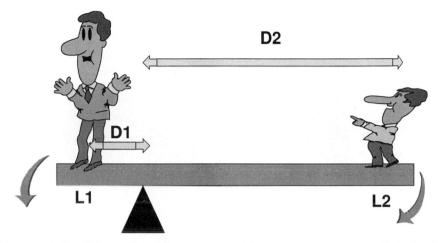

Figure 4–1. Schematic of the moment of force on a teeter-totter. If the load is known in Newtons and the distance in meters, the moment is in newton-meters, or N·m (in the imperial system, the force may be in pounds and the distance in feet, giving a moment in ft-lb). In this case, the same moment about the pivot point (balanced condition) is created by two different weights. In the body, the pivot is an articulation; the short length is typically the distance from the joint to a muscle insertion and the longer length is the distance from the articulation to the load.

close to or far away from the body (with the trunk flexed). Figure 4–3 compares the moment at the lumbar spine (and thus the loads on the lumbar tissues) in the two positions with and without the load in the hands. For comparison, the moments equivalent to the National Institute of Occupational Safety and Health (NIOSH) action limit (AL) and the maximum permissible limit (MPL) are shown. For joint moments below the AL, there is suggested to be minimal risk of low back injury; for values between the AL and MPL, there is increased risk, and above the MPL, there is significantly increased risk of low back injury (NIOSH, 1981; Waters et al., 1993).

The moment is low for upright standing, and even the lifting of the 10-kg load close to the body requires quite small joint moments (loads) at the spine compared to the NIOSH guidelines. Note, however, that flexing forward, even with no load in the hand, requires joint moments close to the recommended AL because of the weight of the torso. The addition of a 10-kg load dramatically increases the low back joint moment, bringing it close to the MPL. This example

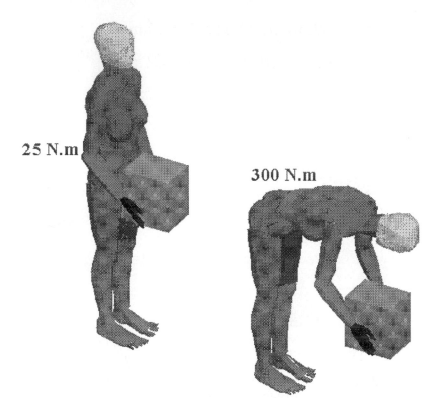

25 N.m

300 N.m

Figure 4–2. The loading on the back, in terms of joint moment, when lifting a 10-kg (~20-lb) load in two different positions, close to or far away from the body. Note that the tissue load is about 12 times greater when bent over. The extensor joint moment indicates that extensor tissues, muscle, and ligament are primarily responsible for maintaining the posture. This demonstrates the importance of how a load is lifted, not just its weight.

illustrates why the weight of an object alone (unless it is extremely heavy) is not a reliable measure of task demand and why the often-heard recommendation for people with low back pain to not to lift more than 20 lb (~10 kg) can either be overprotective (in upright postures with the load close to the trunk) or hazardous (reaching into an automobile to place an 10-kg baby in a car seat), depending on the lifting conditions.

The joint moment of force also explains why even picking up a pencil can induce substantial joint moments with accompanying high muscle/ligament loads. Figure 4–3 shows that the weight of the upper trunk alone can produce substantial loads on the low back if the trunk is flexed so that it lies approximately parallel to the ground. A similar effect can also be seen at the shoulder. The joint moments resulting from body weight have been termed the "hidden load" and

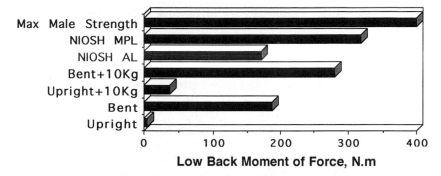

Figure 4–3. Comparison of the moment at the lumbar spine (and thus the loads on the lumbar tissues) in two trunk positions with and without the load in the hands. For comparison, the moment equivalent to the NIOSH action limit (AL) and the maximum permissible limit (MPL) are shown (see text for description). The average maximum strength of men is also indicated for reference.

should always be accounted for whenever the trunk or arm are in nonvertical positions.

Many industries have eliminated the lifting of heavy weights by people in their operations, but, as has been demonstrated above, this does not necessarily mean that the risk factors for low back pain have been eliminated. Reaching away from the body and lifting any load from the floor increases the low back joint moment as a result of both the distance of the load from the body and the "hidden load" of the trunk.

Posture as a Predictor of Tissue Load

Postures of the limbs and trunk have a long history in characterizing tasks because, unlike many other risk factors, they are usually observable and quantifiable without instrumentation. Posture is an important element of task analysis because it can be related to a number of injury mechanisms. In general, posture can give information about four kinds of stressors on the musculoskeletal system (Table 4–2). First, if a limb segment is inclined with respect to the line of gravity, a *joint moment of force* is required about the proximal end, with the necessity for muscular or ligamentous forces to support it. Second, a joint angle close to the end range of motion ("extreme" posture) will load ligaments and may compress blood vessels and nerves. Third, joint angles away from the joint's optimal working range will change the geometry of the muscles crossing the joint and impair the function of joints or of tendons around the joint. Fourth,

TABLE 4–2. Potential Uses of Posture in Task Analysis

Aspect of Posture Observed	Possible Relationship to Musculoskeletal Disorders
Limb segment inclined with respect to the line of gravity	A joint *moment of force* is required with the necessity for muscular or ligamentous forces to support it
A joint angle close to the end range of motion (extreme posture)	Loads ligaments and may compress blood vessels, affect nerves by traction
Joint positions away from the joints' optimal working range	Changes the geometry of the muscles and tendons crossing the joint; may make a given task more fatiguing or stressful
Change (or lack of change) in posture	Characterizes the frequency (repetitiveness) or the static nature of the task

the change (or lack of change) in posture may be used to characterize the frequency (repetitiveness) or the static nature of the task.

Posture as a Predictor of Joint Moment of Force. As the previous section illustrated, the joint moment of force gives important insights into tissue loads. As body segments deviate from the vertical, the ever-present force of gravity acts on the mass of each body segment. The "hidden load" of the arm mass about the shoulder and particularly the trunk mass about the low back is important, especially in sedentary tasks in which the same posture may be maintained for substantial periods of time. This is frequently termed postural load.

"Extreme" Posture as a Predictor of Soft Tissue Loads. Usually the extremes of a joint's motion are constrained by ligaments: Use of extreme posture during work is undesirable. For example, in the low back during "stoop" lifts (where the legs are straight and full flexion of the spine is required), flexion of the lumbar spine creates tension in the posterior ligaments of the spine, and in many people a "flexion relaxation" phenomenon is seen whereby the extensor muscles of the spine become inactive and the ligaments support the moment (McGill and Norman, 1992). The drawback and potential risk in this for low back injury is that, if there are unexpected loads or slipping, the only structures that can support the extra loads are the ligaments. If the posture is held for long periods of time (e.g., in steel reinforcement workers or gardeners), elongation (creep) of the ligament can occur, with a potential reduction in the stability of the spine. (Both of these occupations require, in popular legend, "a cast iron back with a hinge in it.") Compared to muscular control, which can accommodate variation in load and does not creep, ligament load is not a recommended strategy.

Joint Posture and Optimal Musculoskeletal Geometry. For each joint, there is a range of posture that minimizes any adverse features of work and that allows effective force application with minimum fatigue and injury potential. Even before an "extreme" posture is reached, there are changes in the function of the musculoskeletal system that usually make the postures less than optimal and that may elevate tissue loads.

For example, at the wrist, extension of greater than about 30 degrees increases pressure within the carpal tunnel, even in normal people, above 30 mm Hg (Rempel, 1995). This pressure level, if maintained for substantial periods of time, likely decreases microcirculation of the structures in the tunnel, including the median nerve. This may be one of the mechanisms by which work activities cause carpal tunnel syndrome.

Another example at the wrist involves grasping a small object with the wrist in flexion. This can require large effort, and forcing the wrist into maximal flexion will usually cause the object to be dropped. This is the basis of a number of actions in self-defense. This example shows that nonoptimal postures require higher efforts to perform a given task. Large deviation from approximately neutral postures can also affect blood supply. For example, looking upward, as during the picking of fruit, can compromise cerebral blood flow, especially if coupled with neck twist (Sakakibara et al., 1987).

Each joint has an optimal position for different work activities. It is often near the midpoint of the range of motion, but this rule has sufficient exceptions to make it unreliable. For example, the knee functions very well close to the extreme straight position during most locomotor tasks.

Change of Posture. Work involves changes in posture, and the changes can be used to quantify the frequency of movements. Frequency of activity is described further in a later section. If postures do not change for long periods of time, such as shoulder and trunk posture during computer (video display terminal) work, the task may be called static.

Static Efforts and Static Postures

Static efforts, constrained postures, and static postures have been associated with pain, fatigue, and muscle disorders in many studies. If these postures are such as to create sizable joint moments or are extreme postures close to the end range of motion or outside of an optimal range, this is at least understandable because the tissues of the musculoskeletal system are under load—muscle may fatigue and ligament may elongate (creep). It appears, however, that even in low loading situations, such as in the shoulders while working at a video display terminal, static posture can lead to pain and injury. Although the pathophysiology is not completely understood, it appears that even low loads maintained for long periods of time cause slowly recovering disturbances in muscle that lead to pain and dysfunction (Larsson et al., 1988). Identifying the presence of static postures is thus an important part of task analysis. This is true for the low back, because extended periods of time spent sitting (especially if vibration is also present, as during driving) can lead to creep and strain of low back tissues (McGill and Norman, 1992). We can expect higher risk of low back problems in people exposed to this situation, and, for a person with pre-existing back problems, this situation is not likely to lead to a successful return to work. Similarly, working with the arms unsupported in front of the body leads to static load on the tissues of the shoulder/neck region. This will likely aggravate any existing shoulder/neck disorders.

Effect of Frequency

There is an obvious difference between performing an action once and performing the same action continuously over the course of the day. The difference is obvious in the effort required, but there is also a difference in injury potential. The duration or frequency characteristics of tasks typically have been described by the term "repetitiveness." Unfortunately, this work is so often used and overused as to make such terms as "repetitive job" and "highly repetitive" almost meaningless. Usually no clear definition of the term is offered, which compounds the confusion.

In general, the word *repetitive* is used in three main ways. First, it is used as a qualitative term to describe both the high frequency of actions and the sameness or monotony of the job. Second, it has been used to describe fast manual work with little apparent rest between movements. Third, repetitive work can be qualified by such measures as cycle time, number of parts per hour, efforts per hour, or keystrokes per hour.

We know quite a lot about the fatigue of metals and other engineering materials, but for living biologic material, the story is quite a lot more complex. Unless the tissue fails quickly at high loads (typical in trauma but not in many WMSDs, which have a slower onset), the process is a balance between damage and the reparative powers of the body. At higher lifting frequencies, the energy demand can also become prohibitive. Increasing the frequency of a task not only means we perform the activity more often but also means the rest (or recovery time) per effort is reduced. This can be expressed as the ratio of the time of the effort divided by the time for the cycle (work plus rest).

We can gain insight into the magnitude of the effect of frequency from some of the psychophysical experiments performed wherein experienced workers chose what they believed were acceptable loads at different work frequencies. The more frequently a load was lifted, the lighter it had to be to remain acceptable. Figure 4–4 shows the factor by which load must be multiplied for a given lifting frequency to be perceived as requiring the same effort as lifting it once (NIOSH, 1981). As the lifting frequency increases, the acceptable load drops. For example, if 20 kg could be lifted *once per day* with certain posture and other factors, then, for the same lift *every 15 seconds* (4 lifts per minute), a lift mass of 20 kg × 0.85 = 17 kg would be predicted to be still acceptable. It should be noted that some authors believe that, at very high lifting frequencies, this approach overestimates workers' capacities. Using similar methods, the effect of increasing frequency of wrist motion has been recently reported (Snook et al., 1995). Figure 4–5 illustrates the effect of increasing the repetitiveness of the task from 2 per minute to 20 per minute. The force that workers thought they could exert dropped by about one third. On the basis of these data, the effect of frequency is not as great as might be expected.

Psychosocial Factors and Musculoskeletal Disorders

There has been an increasing recognition of the influence of social and psychological factors in the development of a wide range of health outcomes, ranging from sickness/absence to stroke and coronary heart disease. There is some evidence that similar pathways may be involved in musculoskeletal disorders. In the workplace, attention has been devoted to so-called work psychosocial factors, which can be thought of as perceptions of the objective features of the work environment, such as work demand, supervision, work pace, or overtime policies.

One way of describing these factors has been popularized by Karasek and Theorell (1990) in their book *Healthy Work*, in which they classify jobs in terms of dimensions of job demand and decision latitude. A job with high demand and low decision latitude, such as grocery cashier, would be thought of as being a high-strain job. Both high physical and psychosocial demands are associated with increased musculoskeletal disorders; for example, Faucett and Rempel

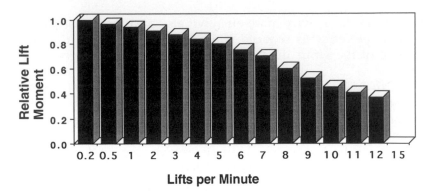

Lifts per Minute

Figure 4–4. Graphic representation of the factor by which a once-per-day lifting effort must be discounted to account for a given lifting frequency. As the lifting frequency increases, the acceptable load drops. (Adapted from National Institute of Occupational Safety and Health: NIOSH Work Practices Guide for Manual Lifting (Technical Report No. 81-122). Cincinnati, OH, U.S. Department of Health and Human Services, 1981.)

(1994) found that, where both factors are present, musculoskeletal disorders are more likely.

TASK ANALYSIS

General Principles

Low Back Demands. For the back, the most important aspects of the job to consider are the maximum moment and the presence of

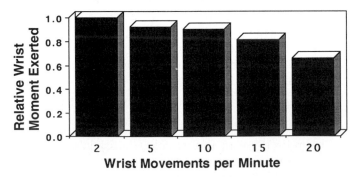

Wrist Movements per Minute

Figure 4–5. Graphic representation of the effect of increasing frequency of wrist motion on acceptable wrist effort. (Adapted from Snook S, Vaillancourt DR, Ciriello VM, et al: Psychophysical studies of repetitive wrist flexion and extension. Ergonomics 38:1488–1507, 1995. Copyright Taylor & Francis Ltd.)

sustained bent or twisted postures. The guidelines in Table 4–3 can be used to identify high-strain work situations for the back.

Shoulder Demands. For the shoulder, the most important aspects of the job to consider are the maximum moment and the presence of elevated arms. Analysis of shoulder demands is heavily based on estimation of moments and observation of posture. Table 4–4 spells out some workplace features useful in analysis.

Hand and Forearm Demands. Analysis of demands on the distal forearm is often more complex than for the shoulder and low back because this area has more kinds of risk factors, the concept of joint

TABLE 4–3. Assessment of Risk Factors for the Low Back*

RISK FACTOR	LOOK FOR
A: High trunk moment; maximum trunk moment is the best single predictor of a high-strain task.	1. Arms reaching forward; the greater the horizontal reach (away from the navel) required to handle a load, the greater the trunk moment. 2. Bent-over trunk posture creating large trunk moments. 3. The weight of the head, arms, and torso. This is half the body weight. It is a hidden, dangerous load. Do not judge manual material handling only by the weight lifted.
B: Nonoptimal postures; spine should be in an optimal posture to support loads.	1. Loss of normal (standing) curve in low back; this indicates the low back is in a nonoptimal posture. 2. Lifting from below knuckle height; forces on spine tissues increases dramatically as a result of large moments and nonoptimal spine postures.
C: Time of loading; vertebral soft tissues (ligaments, muscles, discs) stretch or compress (creep) if loaded for long periods of time, which may lead to instability.	1. Lifting immediately following prolonged immobility without allowing a minute or so for the discs to regain normal size and shape. 2. Sustained or repetitive bent or twisted torso postures, even without high force on the hand. 3. Repeated loading of spinal tissues measured, for example, by total weight lifted. This appears important in low back pain.

*All potential health effects depend on the length of exposure to the conditions, the magnitude or size of the stressor, and the variation of the exposure.

TABLE 4-4. Assessment of Risk Factors for the Shoulder Region*

RISK FACTOR	LOOK FOR
A: High moments at the shoulder	1. The hands far from the body, especially if there is a load in the hands. 2. The arms out from the body or above mid-torso; this puts heavy demand on the neck and shoulder muscles because each arm weighs about 4 kg.
B: Static load on the shoulder girdle; continuous low loads can be as fatiguing and injurious as infrequent high loads.	1. The arms out from the body continuously without support. 2. Shoulder girdle elevation. 3. Tools held continuously.
C: Awkward postures of the shoulder.	1. Work above shoulder level. 2. Work with the arm behind the trunk.
D: No time for recovery of tissues	1. Continuous repetition of the same activity, which may not allow recovery of the involved tissues. 2. More than one third of the person's strength exerted for more than one third of the time; this may lead to incomplete recovery.

*All potential health effects depend on the length of exposure to the conditions, the magnitude or size of the stressor, and the variation of the exposure.

moment is not as easily applied, and movements of the hands may be very rapid. For the hand and forearm, the most important aspects of the job to consider are the maximum force exerted and the frequency of the effort. Table 4-5 shows an approach to analysis of hand and forearm risk factors.

Demands from Sitting and Standing.   Many questions surround the issue of standing and sitting, and so they have been separated from the body region breakdown. In general, sitting and standing have their most direct effect on the low back and the lower limbs. However, inadequate seating can affect the upper limbs. Continuous sitting or standing is likely to lead to problems: a mixture of the two is optimal. Table 4-6 develops an approach to the evaluation of sitting and standing.

General Approach

A structured approach to task analysis is needed so that all necessary information is collected.

TABLE 4–5.   Assessment of Risk Factors for the Hand and Forearm Region*

Risk Factor	Look For
A: High forces and highly repetitive work; these do not mix well.	1. Work with a cycle time of a few seconds. 2. Little "rest" time between cycles (upper limbs in constant motion). 3. Evidence of high forces (see B).
B: Use of high forces; this increases the strain.	1. Use of a pinch grip where a power grasp is more appropriate. 2. Pressing in fasteners with a single finger. 3. Fingers forced into hyperextension. 4. Gloves; these can increase grip force requirements of the task. 5. Lifting in the pronated posture.
C: Nonoptimal postures.	1. Sustained flexion or extension over 30 degrees. 2. Rapid, continuous wrist motions. 3. Sustained ulnar or especially radial deviation. 4. Jerky, flicking, or tossing motions of the wrist. 5. Sustained full pronation.
D: Static loads; should be kept as low as practicable.	1. Gloves; these can create a "static" load on the finger flexors. 2. Holding the wrist in extension, (e.g., during typing); this leads to a "static" load on the finger extensors. 3. Continuously holding a tool or object.
E: Power tools with high vibration, high torques, or poor torque characteristics; these can put heavy demands on the upper limbs.	1. Evidence of "kickback," forcing the wrist rapidly into extension. 2. Vibration of the tool; this can lead to calluses or nerve and blood vessel damage.
F: Sharp edges and hard surfaces; these can lead to calluses or nerve and blood vessel damage.	1. Contact with hard or sharp objects on the sides of the fingers or the base of the palm. 2. Bearing weight on the inside of the elbow on a hard surface. 3. Hammering trim or parts with the palm or "jogging" of paper (striking object with the hand).
G: High-precision placement requirements; these increase time and often force static postures, and risk poor quality.	1. Holding parts stationary to fit them together. 2. Spending time in an awkward posture to thread or fit parts.

*All potential health effects depend on the length of exposure ot the conditions, the magnitude or size of the stressor, and the variation of the exposure.

TABLE 4–6. Assessment of Risk Factors for Sitting and Standing*

Risk Factor	Look For
A: Sitting (see also Table 4–3); standing is better for a variety of tasks with higher forces.	1. Long reaches. 2. Loads over 5 kg (10 lbs). 3. Long periods of sitting (over 1 hr) without an opportunity for standing for a few minutes. 4. Using a chair with inadequate knee room; this is worse than standing.
B: Standing; sitting is better for precision tasks with low force and limited reach requirements.	1. Long periods spent standing (over 1 hr) without taking more than two steps at a time.
C: Incorrect work surface height; this can lead to back, shoulder, neck, or arm fatigue and pain.	1. Too high a work surface, above elbow height and requiring arm abduction. 2. Too low a work surface, below elbow height and requiring the person to stoop over.
D: Poor chair design.	1. Seat too high or sharp edged; this can lead to legs getting tired or swollen, or sore feet. A foot rest is required in this circumstance. 2. A bad or missing back rest; this can lead to a fatigued and stiff back. 3. Lack of adjustability; this makes it difficult to achieve comfort. 4. Four-legged base; this is more likely to tip over than five legs. 5. Arm rests that do not allow the chair to be pulled up close to the work surface.

*All potential health effects depend on the length of exposure to the conditions, the magnitude or size of the stressor, and the variation of the exposure.

Job Description. Task analysis begins with a detailed description of the job. A job description should be obtained from the worker. The analyst must be sure to obtain a complete description in terms of actions, weights, and frequencies of all duties and tasks, even irregular ones, because general descriptions such as "repetitive lifting" or "shipping" or "packing" are of little use.

Ideally, the health care professional will have an opportunity to see the job with the worker concerned performing it. A plain description can be quite misleading. A "sitting job" may range from an almost immobile monitoring task to a sewing job with reaching, twisting, and bending. In addition, all people do not do jobs in the same way. If a personal visit is not practical, a videotape or a physical demand analysis can give excellent insight into the job. If neither of these is available, the job description from the human resources department is a good start.

Task Breakdown. After the job description, the next step is a task breakdown. A task can be considered to be a coherent series of actions to accomplish a goal. Good examples of tasks for a custodian of a school could be mopping floors, emptying mop buckets, polishing floors, and lifting chairs onto tables (see Table 4–7). Notice that the task breakdown will facilitate the description of the physical aspects of the work, because emptying the mop bucket and lifting chairs both involve lifting. This allows the risk factors to be allocated to tasks and may provide a means of changing the person's risk factors by eliminating one task as long as it is not essential to the job. If tasks comprise many different activities, it is probably worth breaking the job down further.

Data Collection. For many industrial jobs, there are a limited number of tasks but they may be repeated many times per shift; for these jobs, information on the frequency or repetitiveness is needed. This can be in the form of production information (e.g., 2,500 units per 8-hour shift). More information must typically be collected on the elements of the tasks performed, especially the forces exerted.

Personnel Input. In addition to the personal investigation described above, there are many who can help in this process of task description and analysis: supervisors, health and safety committee members, industrial engineers, the plant ergonomist, and other work-

TABLE 4–7.   Example Task Breakdown for Custodial Staff

TASK	DURATION OR % TIME	MAJOR RISK FACTORS	CONTRAINDICATIONS
Mopping floors	3 hr/night		
Emptying mop bucket	Twice/night		
Lifting floor polishing machine up a flight of stairs	Once/wk		
Polishing floors	1 hr/night		
Stacking tables and chairs	Once/mo		
Emptying garbage pails in rooms	20 rooms/night		
Wiping boards and tables with cloth	1 hr/night		

ers. Everyone can help identify improvements and get to the root causes of difficulties so that needed changes may be made.

Assessment of Risk Factors in Workplace Tasks

After breaking down the job into coherent tasks, the concepts developed earlier in this chapter can be used to suggest potential risk factors. Using the earlier example of the school custodian, the task analyses described in Tables 4–3 through 4–6 are applied to the task breakdown, as shown in Table 4–8. The relative importance of each risk factor in the development of WMSDs of the different body regions (high, medium, and low) are based on reports in the literature and the experience of the author; the risk in a particular situation may differ depending on equipment, work methods, and the individual concerned.

Depending on method, the first task, mopping floors, will often require working with the arms above shoulder level. The static muscle activity to stabilize the shoulder girdle and move the mop often leads to fatigue in the shoulder region and possible aggravation of pre-existing conditions. Using the mop also requires constant gripping of the mop handle; this may aggravate carpal tunnel syndrome and other disorders of the hand/wrist region. The task is performed every day for about 3 hours, possibly continuously, making these risk factors of medium importance.

The next task, emptying mop buckets into a sink, is a high-risk activity because of the magnitude of the risk factors: high trunk moments and lifting from floor level. In addition, because of the sometimes cramped situations in custodial closets, it is likely that twisted and laterally bent postures are simultaneously present. The presence of high spinal loads and nonoptimal postures to support them is central to assessing the task as high risk despite the relatively low frequency of lifting. Similar arguments can be made for the next task, lifting the floor-polishing machine up a flight of stairs, as well. Here the risk is likely higher. It is likely that, unless detailed questioning is performed, this task will be overlooked by the worker because of its infrequent performance.

The task of floor polishing is usually performed by "locking" the handles of the polisher against the abdomen and controlling the polisher by pivoting the whole trunk; there is no twist in the trunk (the posture is still optimal) but twisting moments are applied to the trunk. The hands typically grip the handles in strong ulnar deviation. The duration is moderate; this leads to a suggestion of low risk for this task.

TABLE 4–8. Example Risk Factor Breakdown for Custodial Staff*

TASK	DURATION OR % TIME	MAJOR RISK FACTORS	CONTRAINDICATIONS
Mopping floors	3 hr/night	Depending on method, working with arms above shoulder level (Table 4–4: C1) Holding mop continuously (Table 4–5: D3)	Shoulder (med) and hand/wrist (low) problems
Emptying mop bucket	Twice/night	High trunk moment (Table 4–3: A1) Lifting from floor level (Table 4–3: B2)	Low back problems (high)
Lifting floor polishing machine up a flight of stairs	Once/wk	High trunk moment (Table 4–3: A1) Lifting from floor level (Table 4–3: B2)	Low back problems (high) and accident risk
Polishing floors	1 hr/night	Awkward wrist posture (Table 4–5: C2) Hand/arm vibration (Table 4–5: E2)	Hand/wrist (low) problems
Stacking tables and chairs	Once/mo	Moderate trunk moment (Table 4–3: A1) Working with arms above shoulder (Table 4–4: C1)	Shoulder and low back problems (low)
Emptying garbage pails in rooms	20 rooms/ night	Lifting from floor level (Table 4–3: A3, B2)	Low back problems (low) Use "golfer's" lift to reach down for pails
Wiping boards and tables with cloth	1 hr/night	Awkward wrist postures (Table 4–5: C1) Working at high levels (Table 4–4: C1) and with extended reaches (Table 4–4: A1)	Wrist, shoulder, and low back problems (med)

*The importance of the risk factor in the development of WMSDs or aggravation of existing WMSDs of the different body regions (high, medium, or low) is based on reports in the literature and the experience of the author; the risk in a particular situation may differ depending on equipment, work methods, and the individual concerned. See text for further explanation

Interested readers are referred to Keyserling et al. (1991) for a description of a structured approach to job analysis.

Some Caveats When Performing a Task Analysis

When looking at jobs to identify risk factors, the health care professional must remember to account for possible effects on workers caused by differences in the time of day and the situation. Not asking questions to identify these effects can mean over-, or more usually under-, estimating the injury potential of the job.

Time Factors.   Risk of back injury increases in the morning or after prolonged sitting, and, as the day progresses, fatigue may set in.

Situational Factors.   Different days or products may offer different demands. A new batch of parts may be more difficult to insert. For high-demand jobs, it may only take a small increase in load to exceed the recuperative powers of the body.

Personal Characteristics.   People differ in many respects, and these differences must be considered. Workers of different height, for example, may need accommodation to get a good match with the job. It is usually better try to change the job rather than select a person who can do it.

WORK MODIFICATION

Although the focus of this chapter is not on work modification, it is worthwhile to make some comments on this topic. In general, ergonomic modifications are divided into two categories: engineering and administrative changes. *Engineering changes* involve physical changes to workstations, products, parts, or tools. Such an approach would modify the custodian's job of emptying mop buckets by installing floor-level drains to allow the bucket to be tipped rather than lifted (this will likely not solve the problem because the work is still performed in a bent-over posture), adding a drain valve or tap, designing a bucket that holds much less water, or installing a powered lift to empty the bucket (unlikely in this situation but common in industrial settings). Note that some of these changes eliminate the risk factors (by emptying with a tap or by powered emptying), whereas others reduce the risk factors (using a smaller bucket).

Administrative changes, by contrast, concentrate on the people and the organization of work. In the custodial example, the administrative changes for emptying the mop bucket could include designating the task "nonessential" to the job and having a co-worker perform it, requiring that full mop buckets be emptied by two people, only performing the task on alternate weeks, or requiring that mop buckets only be half-filled with water. As with engineering changes, some of these may be effective in reducing the risk to the given worker (having a co-worker perform the task), but the risk may now accrue to another worker. The main difficulty with administrative changes is that they may not be adhered to; a rush job will likely mean that the worker cannot wait for a co-worker to help or the co-worker is not available. Because of a change in the worker or the supervisor, the administrative control may be forgotten. Engineering changes, in contrast, tend to be more permanent, affect all workers on that job, and are unlikely to be bypassed under time pressure. For these reasons, engineering changes are usually recommended as a first approach, and only if they cannot be instituted or further risk reduction is required are administrative controls introduced.

A number of conclusions can be drawn from the previous descriptions. Primary prevention is most desirable, but this means that the design of products, tools, and processes must take into account the capabilities of the population. The process of incorporating ergonomics into design is still in its infancy. In general, of the three major classes of risk factors—force, posture, and time (repetition or frequency)—we know least about the effects of time. For primary prevention, on a workstation-by-workstation basis, it is usually easiest to modify postures and force application. These can often be modified with minor effects on production rate (and with a potential for increased productivity). Reducing risk factors associated with time is more difficult. Reducing either frequency of movements or the time spent performing the task per day will usually have a major effect on production; looking at the effect of frequency on moment or weight in Figure 4–4 or Figure 4–5 shows that a very large reduction in frequency is needed to produce marked changes in acceptable force exerted. The number of movements or action *per part* must therefore be reduced; this usually requires product redesign or special tooling, an engineering approach.

If the movement frequency cannot be sufficiently reduced, administrative approaches of short workdays or rotation to other jobs may be a solution. Rotation, the planned movement of a person between a number of jobs, has been adopted widely. In theory, the different jobs in the rotation sequence "dilute" the exposure of any tissue of the back, shoulder, lower limbs, or hands, reducing the risk of developing WMSD. In addition, if job enlargement or enrichment (defining the job with a variety of types of work, such as fetching parts, assembly, packing, and stock ordering) is practiced, the physical and mental challenges are more varied. In practice, it is difficult to find a range of jobs with different demands in many industrial environments, with the result that workers rotate between very similar jobs. Whether this is a useful practice is not known. In addition, there is the justifiable criticism that, if a task within a job is of high risk, rotation may be used to delay proceeding with engineering changes and merely expose extra workers to these stressors.

For return to work of an individual, choice of a "light duty" job or modification of the workstation is usually required. With regard to workstations, posture and force requirements can usually be most easily modified. For selection of "light duty" jobs, it is especially important to examine the available jobs carefully. What to common sense may appear light may be very stressful to a particular worker. A job that can only be done seated and in which breaks are infrequent may appear light but would not be a good choice for many people recovering from low back pain. Likewise, the exhortation not to lift more than 20 lb may exclude a lifting job at waist height with only slow movements but encourage return to a job requiring rapid movements to the floor with light loads.

Acknowledgments. The author would like to acknowledge the input of Robert Norman and Jorma Saari and the staff of the Centre for Occupational Health and Safety, University of Waterloo, into the risk analysis approach incorporated in this chapter.

REFERENCES

Faucett J, Rempel D: VDT-related musculoskeletal symptoms: Interactions between work posture and psychosocial work factors. Am J Ind Med 26: 597–612, 1994.

Frazer TM: Fitness for Work. London, Taylor and Francis, 1992.

Hagberg M, Silverstein B, Wells R, et al (eds): Work-Related Musculoskeletal Disorders (WMSD): A Handbook for Prevention. London, Taylor and Francis, 1995.

Karasek RA, Theorell T: Healthy Work: Stress, Productivity, and the Reconstruction of Working Life. New York, Basic Books, 1990.

Keyserling WM, Armstrong TJ, Punnett L: Ergonomic job analysis: A structured approach for identifying risk factors associated with overexertion injuries and disorders. Appl Occup Environ Hyg 6:353–363, 1991.

Larsson SE, Bengtsson A, Bodegård I, et al: Muscle changes in work related chronic myalgia. Acta Orthop Scand 59:552–556, 1988.

Marras WS, Lavender SA, Leurgans SE, et al: The role of dynamic three-dimensional trunk motion in occupational-related low back disorders: The effects of workplace factors, trunk position and trunk motion characteristics on risk of injury. Spine 18:617–628, 1993.

McGill SM, Norman RW: Low back biomechanics in industry: The prevention of injury through safer lifting. In Grabiner M (ed): Current Issues in

Biomechanics. Champaign, IL, Human Kinetics Publishers, 1992, pp 69–120.

National Institute of Occupational Safety and Health: NIOSH Work Practices Guide for Manual Lifting (Technical Report No. 81-122). Cincinnati OH U.S. Department of Health and Human Services, 1981.

Rempel D: Musculoskeletal loading and carpal tunnel pressure. *In* Gordon S, Blair S, Fine L (eds): Repetitive Motion Disorders of the Upper Extremity. Rosemont, IL, American Academy of Orthopedic Surgeons, 1995, pp 123–133.

Sakakibara H, Miyao M, Kondo T, et al: Relationship between overhead work and complaints of pear and apple orchard workers. Ergonomics *30*:805–815, 1987.

Snook S, Vaillancourt DR, Ciriello VM, et al: Psychophysical studies of repetitive wrist flexion and extension. Ergonomics *38*:1488–1507, 1995.

Waters TR, Putz-Anderson V, Garg A, et al: Revised NIOSH equation for the design and evaluation of manual lifting tasks. Ergonomics *36*:749–776, 1993.

5

Work-Relatedness of Musculoskeletal Disorders

Richard Wells ⸻

Discussions of the association of work with musculoskeletal disorders have had a long history, progressing from observations of patterns of disease among various trades and occupations to more recent studies wherein the "exposure" of individuals to physical and other stresses has been quantified. Precisely because of the controversy over the relationship between work and the causation or aggravation of musculoskeletal disorders, this chapter briefly reviews the epidemiologic, physiologic, and clinical evidence linking these disorders with specific features of work. A task force in the Province of Quebec (including this author) recently reviewed just these issues (Hagberg et al., 1995). Reference to this text will be made for the interested reader.

TERMINOLOGY AND CATEGORIZATION

When exposure to some workplace hazard is directly associated with a given health outcome (such as vinyl chloride with carcinoma), the term "occupational disease" is appropriate. However, when there are multiple factors at work associated with the disease and when even nonwork exposures can produce the disease, then the term "work-related disease" is more appropriate. If the health outcome has a clear pathologic process or agent, then the term "disease" is appro-

TABLE 5–1. Tissue Types and Locations Commonly Included as WMSDs

TISSUE TYPE	EXAMPLE
Tendon	Tenosynovitis, peritendinitis
Muscle	Trapezius or forearm myalgia
Nerve	Carpal tunnel syndrome
Blood vessels	Hypothenar hammer syndrome, Raynaud's disease
Bone, cartilage	Hip or acromioclavicular osteoarthrosis
Unspecified/unknown tissue	Tension neck syndrome (in this example, muscle tissue is likely the cause of symptoms)

priate. However, when some of the outcomes are of uncertain pathogenesis and may consist of symptoms without obvious signs, the term "disorder" is more accurate. For this reason, the outcomes of interest here are termed *work- or activity-related musculoskeletal disorders* (WMSDs).

In general, there are many features of work that are positive, and the working population is generally healthier than the nonworking population. There are, however, negative health outcomes associated with many types of work, and these can be manifested in most organs of the body. Musculoskeletal disorders have achieved increasing recognition over the previous few decades as a range of disorders related to work. Approaches to categorization of nontraumatic injuries, diseases, and disorders of the musculoskeletal system that are observed at work are still in a state of flux, with little agreement on terminology and diagnosis. Table 5–1 suggests one approach to such a categorization.

We may describe the exposure to workplace stressors in many ways, from job categories to detailed descriptions of risk factors. Most current evidence is associated with the physical or biomechanical aspects of the job. Table 5–2 gives examples of the types of physical stressors present at work that have been linked to the development

TABLE 5–2. Biomechanical Risk Factors Commonly Linked to the Development of Musculoskeletal Disorders*

Configuration and arrangement of the environment
Forces exerted
Postures adopted
Frequency and variation in time of forces and postures

*Biomechanical exposures are typically found in work, leisure, and activities of daily living.

of WMSD. However, there is increasing evidence that the psychosocial aspects of work are also important (see Chapter 17). Psychosocial risk factors can be understood as the worker's perceptions of the objective aspects of work organization: the design, pacing, scheduling, and supervision of work.

ELEMENTS OF WORK RELATEDNESS

At work, the musculoskeletal system is acted on by a wide range of factors. Depending on their strength and duration, these stressors may (individually or collectively) lead to changes in musculoskeletal health. Those that cause or aggravate musculoskeletal disorders are known as *risk factors* for WMSD. The relationship between these features of work and the development of WMSD as shown in Figure 5–1, is the focus of this chapter.

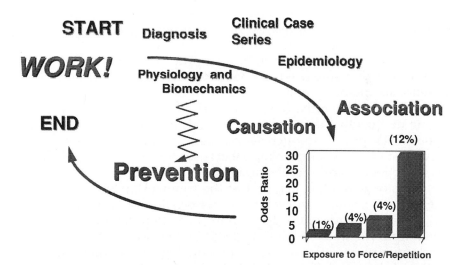

Figure 5–1. Schematic of the interrelationships between work and musculoskeletal disorders. Moving clockwise from WORK, the figure shows how epidemiology is key in demonstrating the association between work and musculoskeletal disorders. The bar chart at the bottom right depicts a typical association between work and musculoskeletal disorders taken from the work of Silverstein (1985). The data are shown enlarged in Figure 5–3 and are further described in the text. Studies of pathophysiology and biomechanics contribute strongly to evidence for causality. Finally, the contribution of epidemiologic and physiologic information to prevention strategy is indicated.

Diagnosis of Disorder

The first step in the picture is the recognition of the presence of musculoskeletal disorders, or *diagnosis*. The approach taken here will be to categorize disorders by tissue type (i.e., muscle, tendon, etc., as well as nonspecific). Table 5–1 illustrates this more fully. In the upper limb, it is often possible to produce a diagnosis to the specific tissue level; however, in the low back, a diagnosis of low back pain is often more appropriate given the uncertainty in specifying the tissue involved (Nachemson, 1992). Other methods of defining the presence of WMSD (the *case definition*) may be based on such actions as filing a compensation claim or self-report of symptoms. In general, the findings of work-relatedness are similar for different case definitions.

Association of Disorder with Work

Clinical case series are often the trigger to consider some feature of work, be it the presence of an organic solvent or the maintenance of stooped work postures, a risk factor for an ill-health outcome. Because the conclusion is based only on the observation of persons with a disorder, this is not a reliable means of determining the work relatedness of a disorder. A well-designed epidemiologic study, however, can reveal the *association* of a disorder with work; that is, the appearance of a suspected risk factor in one group and its relative absence in another group is reflected in different rates of musculoskeletal disorders in the two groups. There are three main epidemiologic designs that are used to assess this association of work relatedness: (1) prevalence (cross-sectional studies), (2) case-control studies, and (3) prospective (or cohort) studies. As we progress from cross-sectional to prospective designs, we allow better control of confounders or biases that may distort the true work relatedness.

Figure 5–1 shows an example of association of work with musculoskeletal disorders; the diagram in the bottom left of the figure is taken from the study of Silverstein (1985) (see also Fig. 5–3). Because a common presentation style for epidemiologic data will be adopted in this chapter, the diagram is briefly described here.

The specific attributes of work studied (work exposures) are indicated along the horizontal axis; in this case, the attributes studied were the combinations of force exerted and the frequency of exertion. Force and frequency were divided into two categories, Hi and Lo. This gives four combinations of work exposure. A cross-sectional study design was used. A large number of workers had their musculoskeletal health—in this case, hand/wrist tendinitis—defined by a physical examination and their exposure to both force and repetition of effort determined. One of the exposure groups, the low-force and low-repetition group (LOF/LOR), was defined as the reference group, and the prevalence of the disorder of interest was compared to this group. This is expressed as the Odds Ratio (OR) for the four groups. The reference group has an OR of 1. If the ORs for the other groups are greater than 1, this implies an association between the different work exposures and the health outcome studied (tendinitis). In the example shown, the ORs increase as we move to high-force and high-frequency (HIF/HIR) tasks, illustrating an association of increased exposure with hand/wrist tendinitis (i.e., work related-ness). Of course, a single study cannot be relied on to determine work relatedness; the accumulation of support from a number of studies is required to affirm this association. Later sections will extend this example to other risk factors and types of disorder.

It is instructive to note the prevalence of (proportion of the group with) hand/wrist tendinitis, shown in brackets above each bar for the different exposure groups. The reference group has a prevalence of 1 per cent, with prevalence rising to 12 per cent in the highest exposure group. Even in the lowest exposure group there are workers with the disorder, and in the highest exposure group not all workers are affected. Moving to higher exposure increases the likelihood of finding hand/wrist tendinitis in the workers. In this discussion we are dealing with the *group of workers*. In examining *an individual* presenting with hand/wrist tendinitis, it is impossible to attribute the condition to work in that individual, although this is more likely if the worker is a member of a high-exposure group.

Causation of Disorders

Even a well-designed prospective study, while allowing inference about the work relatedness of a particular risk factor for WMSD, only provides a part of the evidence needed to address *causation* of musculoskeletal disorders. The other part of the picture of causation comes from the synthesis of biologic, physiologic, and clinical information. This route addresses the causal mechanisms of WMSD. For example, it has been shown that working with the wrist in even moderate flexion or extension elevates the intracarpal pressure to above 30 mm Hg. That is a level that will promote ischemic conditions in the contents of the carpal canal. If this position is maintained for long periods of time, as when performing data entry tasks, there is a likelihood of inducing symptoms of carpal tunnel syndrome. The support of epidemiologic studies by laboratory evidence increases our confidence that work is not only associated with WMSD but is also causative.

Another purpose for the study of causation of musculoskeletal disorders is that such knowledge can inform both treatment and prevention activities. Better knowledge of injury mechanisms may provide better treatment decisions. For example, recent data on the pressure in the carpal canal at different functional wrist angles has demonstrated that the pressure is lowest in neutral and rises sharply with extension. A common prescription for conservative treatment of carpal tunnel symptoms is a "cock-up" night splint, which places the wrist in moderate extension. This contradiction has recently been clinically explored, and a neutral night splint (which we expect to have smaller carpal canal pressures) has been found to produce more relief of symptoms than the traditional extension splint (Burke et al., 1994).

Investigation of causality may also lead to better interventions in the workplace to prevent the development of WMSD. The epidemiologic investigation provides associations between risk factors and WMSD. Because these investigations require moderately large numbers of participants, it is difficult to collect detailed information on the work; we must usually be content with descriptions of work that quantify for example, "use or not of a computer mouse" or "VDT work of over 4 hours' duration per day." This provides impetus for control of these risk factors by elimination or reduction of the risk factor concerned. However, data must still be entered into computers; we cannot reduce the time spent working at computers to zero. Therefore, information on *why* use of a computer mouse may cause WMSD or what aspects of computer use may lead to WMSD is critical in the design of new data entry methods.

DOCUMENTATION OF WORK RELATEDNESS

Occupational epidemiologists have developed a list of criteria to help assess the validity of inferences of association and causation between work and adverse health outcomes; these include whether there are a number of studies showing the same effect, how strong the relationships are, whether the cause occurs before the effect, and whether there is a plausible biologic pathway between the cause and the effect.

The framework often used in epidemiology for assessment of causality is used here to present a range of evidence concerning work relatedness. These criteria are described and summarized in Table 5–3. Fuller details of the studies of the work relatedness of muscu-

TABLE 5-3. Criteria for Assessing Work Relatedness and Causality

CRITERION	DESCRIPTION	NOTES
Is there an association between features of work and a musculoskeletal disorder?	Are there flaws in the studies?	Evaluation of individual epidemiologic studies is outside the scope of this work; see, for example, Bombardier et al. (1994)
	What is the strength of the relationship?	
	Is there an exposure-response relationship?	Do higher levels of the risk factor give higher levels of the disorder (higher incidence or prevalence)?
Is there consistency?	Do a number of studies have similar findings?	See Stock (1991) and Hagberg et al. (1995)
Is there a temporal relationship? Do changes in work exposures result in a change in disorders?	Does the effect (musculoskeletal disorders) occur after the cause (work)?	This is difficult to assure in cross-sectional and case-control designs; prospective studies offer the best evidence
Does the association agree with other evidence?	Is the association biologically, clinically, or physiologically plausible?	For a review, see Hagberg et al. (1995)

loskeletal disorders and pathophysiologic pathways can be found in Hagberg et al. (1995) and Gordon et al. (1995).

Evidence of Consistent Association

The first epidemiologic criteria for assessment of work relatedness of WMSD are whether there is an association between features of work and a musculoskeletal disorder, and whether there is consistency in that association. Do a number of studies have similar findings, and what is the strength of the relationship? A large number of studies have examined the association of work with musculoskeletal disorders (Hagberg et al., 1995). The studies are presented by the type of tissue affected: tendon, nerve, and unspecified.

TENDON-RELATED DISORDERS

In most studies, cases of tendinitis and tenosynovitis have been defined based on physical examination. Studies have been performed in both the shoulder and hand/wrist region. Figure 5–2 illustrates a typical study of the association of overhead work with shoulder tendinitis (Bjelle et al., 1979).

Figure 5–3 shows an example of an exposure-response relationship between hand/wrist tendinitis and the forcefulness and frequency of efforts (Silverstein, 1985). As the work exposure moves from low force to high force and low repetition to high repetition, the risk of disorders increases.

Tendon-related disorders in both the hand and the shoulder have demonstrated a moderate to strong and consistent relationship with various risk factors at work. In the shoulder region, overhead work appears as a strong risk factor, whereas, in the hand, forces and frequency of effort have been most commonly identified.

NERVE-RELATED DISORDERS

Although carpal tunnel syndrome has been extensively studied, a number of other sites of entrapment have been studied less. Case definitions have been based on electrodiagnostic studies, symptom reports (usually pain and numbness or nocturnal tingling), physical

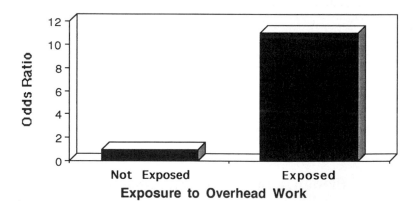

Figure 5–2. Example of the relationship between work exposure and shoulder tendinitis. Seventeen workers with degenerative shoulder tendinitis were matched with 34 workers from the same workshops and of the same age (case-control design). Work was classified as above or below shoulder level based on worksite observation. (Adapted from Bjelle A, Hagberg M, Michaelsson G: Clinical and ergonomic factors in prolonged shoulder pain among industrial workers. Scand J Work Environ Health 5:205–210, 1979.)

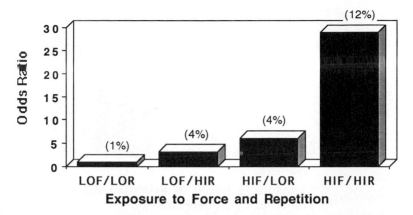

Figure 5–3. Example of an exposure-response relationship between work exposure and hand and wrist tendinitis. A cross-sectional study design with 574 male and female workers was used. The presence of hand and wrist tendinitis was defined by a physical examination. Exposure to force and repetition of effort was determined by measurement and observation. Force and frequency were divided into two categories, Hi and Lo. (Adapted from Silverstein BA: The prevalence of upper extremity cumulative trauma disorders in industry. Doctoral thesis, University of Michigan, Ann Arbor, 1985.)

examination using a variety of tests (often Phalen's or Tinel's), or a combination of all these methods. Similar associations with work are found, irrespective of whether electrodiagnostic or symptom-based case definitions are used.

Studies of work exposures have concentrated on vibration, forceful exertions, pinch grips, and non-neutral work postures. An example is seen in Figure 5–4 of a strong association found between long periods of time spent flexed or extended postures at work and carpal tunnel syndrome defined electrodiagnostically (de Krom et al., 1990).

UNSPECIFIED/UNKNOWN TISSUE DISORDERS

In many cases, it is not possible to identify pain and discomfort as emanating from a particular tissue. These disorders are often described as nonspecific, although in some common disorders, such as tension neck syndrome, muscle tissue is suspected of being involved.

Figure 5–5 shows an example of an exposure-response relationship between upper limb pain and discomfort, and different heights of the worker's computer keyboard (Bergqvist et al., 1995). As the keyboard is raised above elbow height, the risk of suffering shoulder and neck problems increases. Conversely, as the keyboard is lowered below elbow height, the risk of developing shoulder/neck problems decreases but the risk of developing hand/arm symptoms increases.

An important class of nonspecific disorders is low back pain. Ex-

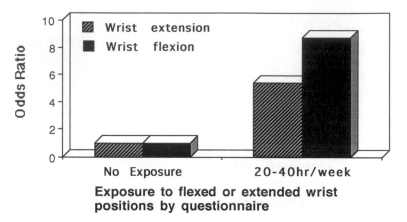

Figure 5–4. Example of a relationship between work exposure and carpal tunnel syndrome. A total of 156 cases of carpal tunnel syndrome were compared with 310 noncases from the same community and were assessed electrodiagnostically. Work exposures were assessed by telephone questionnaire. (Adapted from de Krom MCTFM, Kester ADM, Knipschild PG, et al: risk factors for carpal tunnel syndrome. Am J Epidemiol 132:1102–1110, 1990.)

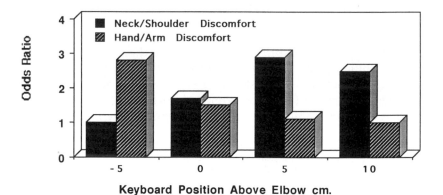

Figure 5–5. Example of an exposure-response relationship between work exposure and pain and discomfort in the upper limbs. This was a cross-sectional study of 260 video display terminal workers. Musculoskeletal pain was assessed by a standardized questionnaire. Ergonomic factors were assessed by worksite observation. Note that, as the keyboard is raised, shoulder pain increases, probably because this forces shoulder abduction and elevation. As the keyboard is lowered, hand and arm discomfort increases, perhaps because more wrist extension is required. (Adapted from Bergqvist U, Wolgast E, Nilsson B, Voss M: Musculoskeletal disorders among visual display terminal workers: individually, ergonomic and work organizational factors. Ergonomics 38:763–776, 1995. Copyright Taylor & Francis Ltd.)

cept in a minority of cases, the tissues involved cannot be determined. Reported cases (to compensation systems) are often used as case definitions. Figure 5–6 illustrates the exposure-response relationship for low back pain cases with increasing levels of awkward postures for the back (Punnett et al., 1991). It can be seen that, even with short periods of time spent in twisted and bent postures, the risk of low back pain for workers increases substantially over that for workers able to spend all their time in an optimal upright position.

An example of the association of the dynamic aspects of work and low back pain and disability is depicted in Figure 5–7 (Marras et al., 1993). Here the factors of maximum trunk moment (weight lifted multiplied by the distance of the weight out from the back) trunk velocity, and weight handled all elevated the risk to the low back.

Evidence of Cause-Effect Relationship

Another epidemiologic criterion for work relatedness is whether there is a temporal relationship and whether changes in work exposures result in a change in disorders. In other words, does the effect (musculoskeletal disorders) occur after the cause (work)? It is difficult to be sure that risk factors at work preceded the development of musculoskeletal disorder in cross-sectional and case-control designs. In both of these types of study, the work exposure is measured at the

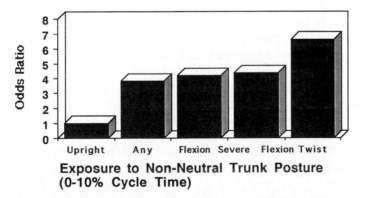

Exposure to Non-Neutral Trunk Posture (0-10% Cycle Time)

Figure 5–6. Example of an exposure-response relationship between work exposure and low back pain in workers with 95 low back pain and 124 controls. Low back pain was indicated by report and physical examination. Work exposure was characterized by transcription of trunk posture from slow-motion videotape. The likelihood of low back pain increases as workers spend time in increasingly more forward-bent and twisted positions. (Adapted from Punnett L, Fine LJ, Monroe W, et al: Back disorders and nonneutral trunk postures of automobile assembly workers. Scand J Work Environ Health 17:337–346, 1991.)

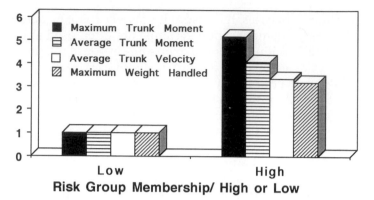

Figure 5–7. Example of an association between the dynamic aspects of work and risk of low back pain. A total of 235 jobs were selected as low or high risk based on reported injuries, turnover, and accident reports. Low-risk jobs had no reported injuries or turnover in the last 3 years. The demands of each job were quantified dynamically using a goniometer attached to the low back as well as by measurement of the dimensions of the workstation and of the weights handled. (Adapted from Marras WS, Lavender SA, Leurgans S, et al: The role of dynamic three-dimensional trunk motion in occupationally-related low back disorders. Spine *18*:617–628, 1993.)

same time as health status. This drawback can be reduced by taking care to make sure, for example, that the onset of the disorder occurred in the current job and that the worker has been on the current job for at least 6 months. This precaution is commonly a part of participant recruitment in prevalence studies. However, a cohort study is the best design for assuring this.

Perhaps the clearest illustration of this type of evidence was found in a study of fish-processing workers by Brubaker et al. (1990). The work is seasonal and the season is short, with long shifts. In addition, the work is performed at high speed and involves forceful manual activities. The research of Silverstein (1985) would suggest that this type of work had a high risk for a number of musculoskeletal disorders of the hand and wrist. The musculoskeletal health status of these workers was determined by physical examination and electro-diagnostic studies of the median nerve both preseason and 30 days after the start of the season. A control group of office staff was also used for comparison (Brubaker et al., 1991). The results for carpal tunnel syndrome are illustrated in Figure 5–8. There was an increase in the risk of developing carpal tunnel syndrome between the beginning of the season and approximately 1 month later. Not only does this satisfy the temporality criterion, but it also shows that a change

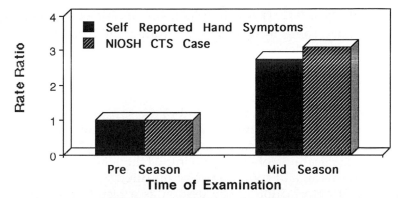

Figure 5–8. Illustration of the temporality criterion wherein work exposures preceded development of carpal tunnel syndrome. A group of seasonal
fish-processing workers had electrodiagnostic studies performed on the median nerve prior to the start of the fishing season and 30 days into the season.
The work was characterized by high-frequency and high-force exertion to
remove the roe from fish. An age-matched group of office workers from the
same plant was used for comparison. (Adapted from Brubaker R, Hertzman
C, Jin A, et al: Prevalence of Muscle, Tendon and Nerve Compression Disorders in the Hand and Wrist of Roe Production Workers in Fish Processing
Plants. Vancouver, Joint Committee of the Fish Processor Association and the
United Fishermen's and Allied Workers Union, and Division of Occupational
and Environmental Health, Department of Health Care and Epidemiology,
University of British Columbia, 1990.)

in work intensity, from low- to high-stress work, results in an increase
in disorders.

Evidence of Pathophysiologic Mechanisms

A final epidemiologic criterion for work relatedness is whether the
association agrees with other evidence (i.e., whether the association
is biologically, clinically, or physiologically plausible). In general,
plausible mechanisms exist for the physical aspects of work to both
cause and aggravate a wide range of musculoskeletal disorders. Because musculoskeletal disorders are associated with work exposures,
these are, by and large, submaximal and do not typically produce
observable effects on the musculoskeletal system quickly. This makes
testing of pathophysiologic mechanisms challenging. Although there
have been some attempts to produce these disorders in animals using
work exposures, most of our knowledge is based on extrapolation
from acute (short-duration) experiments in volunteers and study of

people with disorders. There are thus many questions remaining unanswered concerning mechanisms of work-related musculoskeletal disorders. The evidence from these studies is presented by type of tissue affected: tendon, nerve, and muscle.

TENDON DISORDERS

Disorders of tendon (tendinitis) and of the surrounding sheath (tenosynovitis) may result from a number of mechanisms at work. Proposed mechanisms of injury include permanent deformation as a result of mechanical microfailure, fraying of the tendon as a result of rubbing and wear, and compromise of nutrition.

Permanent deformation of the tendon as a result of sustained or repeated submaximal loads has been suggested as leading to an inflammatory response. Testing on cadaveric tendon has indicated that a plausible history of loading, typical of industrial tasks, can produce such a deformation. This has been termed a cumulative strain in the tendon.

Work exposures may also lead to degeneration of the tendon; for example, in the shoulder there is a region of potential avascularity of the supraspinatus tendon in the region of the head of the humerus. Degeneration results from impairment of blood flow coupled with mechanical stress. Impairment of blood flow is likely during overhead work or arm abduction. This results from the high internal pressure generated within the supraspinatus muscle, which will tend to impede the blood supply to the tendon running through the muscle. Direct mechanical stress is possible in this region because the rotator cuff tendons may become trapped against the coracoacromial arch during elevation of the arm (impingement).

NERVE DISORDERS

Nerve tissue can be injured or irritated by elevated hydrostatic pressure, mechanical contact, or stretch. Most information is available about the median nerve within the carpal canal, on which cadaveric studies as well as tests in volunteers have been performed. The action of elevated hydrostatic pressure and mechanical contact stress is discussed here. Although stretching of nerves in the production of nerve disorders has some support from an animal model, it will not be discussed further.

Application of external pressure over the carpal has been shown to raise intracarpal pressures. At some critical pressure between 30 and 60 mm Hg, symptoms mimicking those of carpal tunnel syndrome (i.e., progressive sensory loss, then motor loss) have been shown to take place over minutes and hours. The apparent mechanism is ischemia of the median nerve tissue. The blood pressure in the capillary bed is approximately 30 mm Hg, supporting this suggestion. In vivo measurements of carpal tunnel pressures in normal persons have demonstrated that functional extended (and to a lesser extent flexed) wrist positions, commonly observed in occupational settings, can elevate intracarpal tunnel pressures above 30 mm Hg. If the length of exposure is sufficient (e.g., sitting at a computer terminal for 7 hours per day), it is plausible that damage to the median nerve can be caused.

Mechanical contact stresses have also been demonstrated in the carpal canal. Cadaver tests have shown that flexed wrist postures combined with pinching or gripping trap the median nerve between the tendons and the flexor retinaculum. This action is the basis of the modified Phalen's test, whereby a pinch grip with a flexed wrist posture is adopted that aggravates any disorders of the median nerve. It is therefore very reasonable to conclude that work activities that involve gripping with a flexed wrist could aggravate or cause carpal tunnel syndrome. If movement of the wrist occurs simultaneously, the likelihood of mechanical damage is heightened.

MUSCLE DISORDERS

There are a number of proposed physiologic mechanisms for muscle disorders, including the manner in which muscle fibers are recruited, motor control, the stresses and pressures generated within muscle during contraction, and disturbances of local circulatory and metabolic conditions.

Control of the amount of force generated by a muscle is determined by the number of muscle fibers activated; this recruitment of additional fibers, or more properly motor units, is always in the same order, from smallest to largest. Low forces will always recruit the small motor units with small fibers, and long-term, low-level contractions will mean that the smallest muscle fibers are continuously active. This is termed static load. Although the muscle as a whole is not overloaded, the small motor units, dubbed "Cinderella" motor units, may become fatigued and suffer damage.

When a muscle is activated, its force production increases and an intramuscular pressure is generated. Even at low force levels, this pressure affects blood flow; the impact on blood flow depends on the muscle considered. For example, the supraspinatus muscle is enclosed in a bony channel, and even moderate abduction or flexion of the arm increases intramuscular pressure above that of the local blood pressure, with potential for damage if this condition continues for extended periods of time.

Disturbances to metabolic conditions are more complex than the mechanisms discussed above, and a full discussion can be found in Chapter 3.

Summary

For some tissues and disorders, there is good evidence that work exposures are associated with the development of injury and that the relative risk of certain work exposures is high; this is true for shoulder and hand/wrist tendinitis, carpal tunnel syndrome, and hypothenar hammer syndrome. In addition, there are a large number of studies that link localized musculoskeletal symptoms of pain and discomfort (e.g., tension neck syndrome and low back pain). In addition to the presence of a consistent *association* between workplace factors and the development of a variety of musculoskeletal disorders, there are plausible biologic pathways by which the physical stresses at work could *cause* these disorders.

REFERENCES

Bergqvist U, Wolgast E, Nilsson B, Voss M: Musculoskeletal disorders among visual display terminal workers: Individually, ergonomic and work organizational factors. Ergonomics 38:4:763–776, 1995.

Bjelle A, Hagberg M, Michaelsson G: Clinical and ergonomic factors in prolonged shoulder pain among industrial workers. Scand J Work Environ Health 5:205–210, 1979.

Bombardier C, Kerr MS, Shannon HS, Frank JW: A guide to interpreting epidemiologic studies on the etiology of back pain. Spine 19(Suppl 18): 2047S–2056S, 1994.

Brubaker R, Hertzman C, Jin A, et al: Prevalence of Muscle, Tendon and Nerve Compression Disorders in the Hand and Wrist of Roe Production Workers in Fish Processing Plants. Vancouver, Joint Committee of the Fish Processor Association and the United Fishermen's and Allied Workers Union, and Division of Occupational and Environmental Health, Department of Health Care and Epidemiology, University of British Columbia, Vancouver, 1990.

Burke D, McHale Burke M, Stewart GW, et al: Splinting for carpal tunnel syndrome: In search of the optimal angle. Arch Phys Med Rehabil 75: 1241–1244, 1994.

de Krom MCTFM, Kester ADM, Knipschild PG, et al: Risk factors for carpal tunnel syndrome. Am J Epidemiol 132:1102–1110, 1990.

Gordon SC, Blair SV, Fine LJ (eds): Repetitive Motion Disorders of the Upper Extremity. Rosemont, IL, American Academy of Orthopaedic Surgeons, 1995.

Hagberg M, Silverstein B, Wells R, et al: Kourinka I, Forcier L (eds): Work Related Musculoskeletal Disorders (WMSDs): A Reference Book for Prevention. London, Taylor and Francis, 1995.

Marras WS, Lavender SA, Leurgans S, et al: The role of dynamic three-dimensional trunk motion in occupationally-related low back disorders. Spine 18:617–628, 1993.

Nachemson AL: Newest knowledge of low back pain: A critical look. Clin Orthop Rel Res 8:279, 1992.

Punnett L, Fine LJ, Monroe W, et al: Back disorders and nonneutral trunk postures of automobile assembly workers. Scand J Work Environ Health 17:337–346, 1991.

Silverstein BA: The prevalence of upper extremity cumulative trauma disorders in industry. Doctoral thesis, University of Michigan, Ann Arbor.

Stock S: Workplace ergonomic factors and the development of musculoskeletal disorders of the neck and upper limbs: A meta-analysis. Am J Ind Med 19:87–107, 1991.

6
Pain Perception

Pain is associated with injury . . . usually but not always. Many are the stories of heroes who have walked through an emotionally charged and dangerous situation with a stable lower limb fracture, without feeling pain at that time. However, pain, especially chronic pain, can also be present, and even severe, because injury was thought to have occurred when in fact it had not (Helme el al., 1990). What, then, is pain?

Pain has been compared to an alarm bell ringing in the conscious mind, alerting us to the *probability* of injury. Its relationship to injury is an indirect one. When we touch a hot stove, we feel pain, but only after the hand has been withdrawn from danger. Tissue injury and the reflex responses of muscles to injury operate at one level. At a higher level, pain is perceived as this lower level stimulus reaches consciousness. There, it is modifiable by high-level influences, both conscious and subconscious (Fig. 6–1).

In 1644, after examining nerve filaments in the bodies he had dissected anatomically, Descartes suggested that, when tissue is damaged, these "delicate threads" mechanically transmit information to the brain "just as by pulling at one end of a rope one makes a bell which hangs at the other end to strike at the same instant" (Wall and Jones, 1991). Neuroanatomists and pain psychologists since that day have done much to deepen our understanding of pain pathways and neurophysiology, but this simple understanding of a direct relationship between pain and injury persists in the public mind. In 1986,

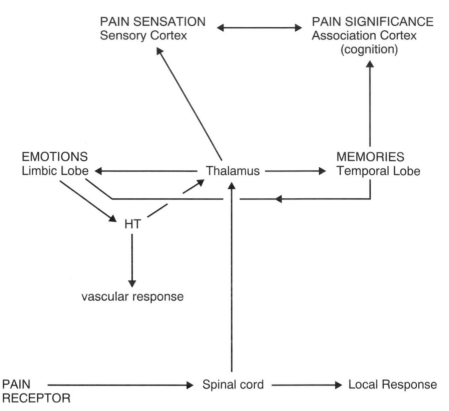

Figure 6–1. Pain signal from periphery interacts with higher centers in the brain that interpret and modify the pain experience. HT = hypothalamus.

Merskey defined pain as "an unpleasant sensory and emotional experience associated with actual or potential tissue damage, or described in terms of such damage." This definition has now been accepted by the International Association for the Study of Pain (IASP) (Merskey and Bogduk, 1994, p. 210).

Although we may think and talk of pain as a sensation, it differs markedly from what we normally consider sensation. It is not so much a sensation as a perception (Morris, 1991, p. 75). A sensor provides information about reality, the validity of this information being proportional to the quality of the sensor. For example, when presented with a hammer, we can see its shape and color, feel its weight, and determine whether it is hot or cold. By deductive reasoning based on data in our memories, we can tell whether the handle is made of wood and the head of iron. These are all characteristics of the hammer; these are properties resident in the hammer that we can sense through our sense organs.

If one strikes one's thumb with the hammer, one will experience pain. Pain is not a property resident in the hammer. It is, rather, an individual's perception regarding an event that has taken place within his or her body. For most people in most situations, that perception will be one of pain. Fitzgerald and Woolf (cited in Chahl et al., 1984, p. 130) have hypothesized that the small, unmyelinated C fibers are actually sensing chemical changes in the tissues following trauma. It is the central nervous system that then interprets this information as pain, and the result of injury. These C fibers, as well as A delta fibers that respond in a similar fashion, are therefore called nociceptive fibers (*nocere*, to injure).

ELEMENTS OF THE PAIN RESPONSE

During the past five decades, we have come to realize that pain perception is an exceedingly complex phenomenon. Because of the many neuroanatomic and neurochemical[1] interactions involved, we can no longer directly relate the intensity of the hurt one feels to the degree of harm that has occurred. What is pain to one person may only be discomfort to another with the same injury. To understand why, let us consider first the local factors initiating the pain response, which give rise to what is known as peripheral pain, and then the central factors that modify the pain experience.

Local Factors: Tissue Response

Tissue damage results in release of intracellular potassium ions, bradykinin, histamine, serotonin, proteolytic enzymes, and arachidonic acid. The latter may then be converted into prostaglandins, thromboxane, and/or leukotrienes (Granström, 1983). Prostaglandins cause pain indirectly by sensitizing nerve endings and producing swelling as a result of the effect of bradykinin. Vasodilation occurs. Hyperalgesia may result. Vasoconstriction may be induced by thromboxane, and leukotrienes may contribute to the development of trigger points. Calcium ions, which are also released from damaged tissue, combine with adenosine triphosphate to produce uncontrolled muscle contractions (Rosomoff, 1985).

Further complicating the situation at the peripheral level is the fact

---

[1]The neurochemistry of pain is a rapidly developing and complex subject that will not be dealt with here. Three references are provided in the Suggested Reading lists for those interested: Duggan and Furmidge (1994), Richardson (1990), and Terenius (1992).

that substance P, a dorsal horn neurotransmitter produced by nociceptive fibers in peripheral nerves, may also be released peripherally into the inflamed area. (For a detailed description of the process of neurogenic inflammation, see Chahl et al., 1984.) This would further increase the degree of inflammation and widen the area involved.

With acute injuries, the tissue response usually resolves in days or weeks but, in a small proportion of these, and in situations in which there is repetitive trauma, hyperalgesia may develop. Repetitive stimulation has long been known to decrease the sensory threshold of nociceptor fibers (Bessov and Perl, 1969). *Hyperalgesia* is an "increased response to a stimulus that is normally painful" (Merskey and Bogduk, 1994, p. 211). It has also been defined as "a state of long-lasting, *post-stimulus* sensory disturbance which is characterized by a *decrease in sensory threshold, increased pain* to suprathreshold stimuli and, often, *ongoing pain after the stimulus has been removed*" (Helme et al., 1990, p. 401). Thus the pain can be greater than one might expect and can persist after the injury should have healed. It is this kind of condition that exists in people with chronic nonmalignant pain.

Furthermore, the area of tenderness may not be confined to the injured area, but may in time extend into the adjacent uninjured tissues. When there is pain in such areas, this has been called "secondary hyperalgesia," but the term "allodynia" is now preferred. The IASP has defined *allodynia* as "pain due to a stimulus that does not normally provoke pain" (Merskey and Bogduk, 1994, p. 211). In animals with chronic arthritic pain, structural alterations have been shown to occur within the spinal cord that expand the area of pain sensitivity (Hylden et al., 1989). This is one possible explanation for allodynia.

Central Factors: Anatomic Pathways

Heat, certain chemical changes within the tissues, and, when tissues are sensitized, even touch, pressure, and movement can generate an electrical response in small myelinated A delta fibers and in even smaller unmyelinated (therefore slow-conducting) C fibers. These transmit pain information to an ascending pathway in the spinal cord, which will ultimately lead to a consciousness of pain. However, A beta and sympathetic fibers can also be involved. Of all of these, most is known about the C fibers.

Pain fibers terminate in the dorsal horn of the spinal cord, where they connect with the two primary ascending pain pathways (Fig. 6–2). At these connections (synapses), chemicals are released by incoming pain fibers that stimulate an electrical discharge in the next neuron in the pathway toward conscious perception. However, the

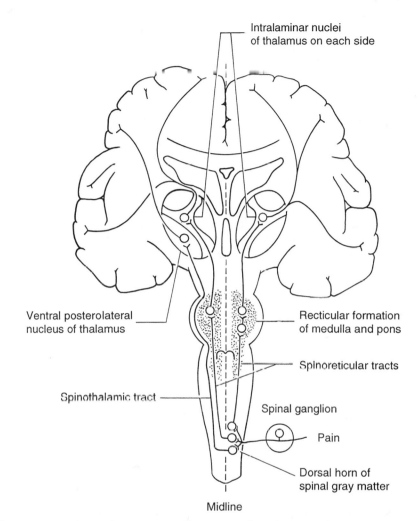

Figure 6–2. Ascending pain pathways within the central nervous system that are well accepted as being important in humans are the spinothalamic, a one-sided (but crossed) pathway for discriminative aspects of the brain, and the spinoreticulothalamic, a bilateral pathway that distributes pain information widely throughout the brain and is concerned with emotional aspects of pain.

mere fact that there is a connection between neurons means that other influences can operate either to facilitate pain signal transmission or to inhibit it. These influences are chemical in nature, primarily coming from other nerves that end here. Some of these descend from higher brain centers. Some, coming in through peripheral nerves, compete with nociceptor signals for a chance to ascend to consciousness. The discovery of such competition has given rise to the concept of a "pain gate." More will be said about this concept later.

The first *ascending pain pathway* to be recognized was the lateral spinothalamic tract. The fibers of this tract cross over the midline and ascend to the brain as a bundle just posterior to the anterior roots of the spinal nerves, close to the surface of the spinal cord. Cutting this bundle was found to eradicate pain in patients with severe pain resulting from inoperable cancer. This result seemed to confirm Descarte's pain theory, but the pain often returned. One reason is that not all the spinothalamic pain fibers are gathered together in the same place. Another reason is that there are other pain pathways.

It used to be taught that all pain fibers were in this lateral spinothalamic tract and that simple touch fibers were in the anterior spinothalamic tract, a bundle located medial to the anterior spinal nerve roots. Although this is to a large extent true, the fact is that these two bundles (pain and temperature in one, simple touch in the other) are somewhat intermixed. So many neuroanatomy texts do not now differentiate between anterior and lateral spinothalamic pathways, simply referring to the combination as the *spinothalamic tract*. This crossed pathway synapses in the caudal part of the ventral posterolateral thalamic nucleus. Fibers from this nucleus carry information about the location of all trunk and limb pain to the sensory cortex on the opposite side of the body. This is where all other general sensory information about that side of the body goes. So, for example, pain from the right hand is projected to the sensory area for the hand in the left parietal cortex. Information about pressure and conscious position sense also reaches this area through other pathways. All of this is *discriminative* information about that particular part of the body.[2]

The other of the two primary pain pathways ascending in the spinal cord is the *spinoreticulothalamic tract* (Fig. 6–2). It ascends in the spinal column intermixed with spinothalamic fibers, and, after synapsing in the brain stem reticular formation, it proceeds to the thalamus. It differs from the spinothalamic tract in important ways anatomically and functionally. First, it ascends bilaterally in the cord and therefore reaches the thalamus of *both* halves of the brain. There it terminates primarily on the intralaminar nuclei of the thalamus. Second, these nuclei then project widely to many areas of cerebral cortex, including the limbic cortex, which is concerned with *emotion*. Thus the spinoreticulothalamic pathway is involved in how we feel about our pain, as opposed to where it is. Thus we have *one pathway*

---

[2]The pain fibers in the head and upper segment of the neck that would correspond to those in the spinothalamic tract travel in the trigeminothalamic tract. Their thalamic destination is similar to that for the spinothalamic tract except that they terminate in the caudal part of the adjacent ventral postero*medial* (not posterolateral) thalamic nucleus.

for sensory-discriminative aspects of pain and another for affective-motiva-tional aspects (Melzack and Casey, 1968).

This second pathway (spinoreticulothalamic) has many more con-nections along the way. Some of these are with the raphe nuclei and the periaqueductal gray matter in the brain stem. From these and other areas, pathways *descend* to the dorsal horn that are capable of modifying reception of various types of sensory input coming in from the periphery. Many influences come from the cerebral cortex itself, including one coming indirectly from the discriminative sensory cor-tex of the contralateral parietal lobe (Fig. 6–3). It is through descend-ing pathways (feedback loops) such as these that the cognitive and

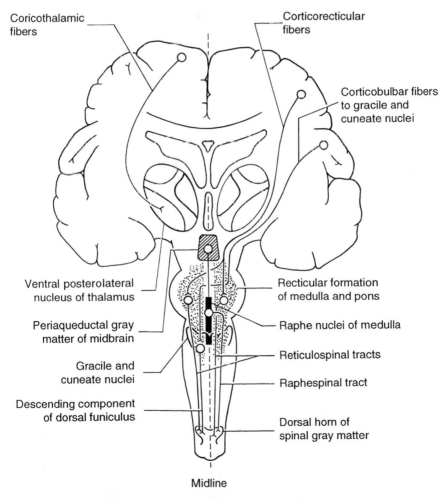

Coricothalamic fibers

Corticorecticular fibers

Corticobulbar fibers to gracile and cuneate nuclei

Ventral posterolateral nucleus of thalamus

Recticular formation of medulla and pons

Periaqueductal gray matter of midbrain

Raphe nuclei of medulla

Gracile and cuneate nuclei

Reticulospinal tracts

Descending component of dorsal funiculus

Raphespinal tract

Dorsal horn of spinal gray matter

Midline

Figure 6–3. Descending pathways that modify sensory input.

emotional influences of the brain can modify sensory input to the spinal cord, giving some credibility to the expression "mind over matter."

It would be wonderful if the human brain could be this simple, but that is not the case.[3] (For those wanting more information, a list of useful books and articles is found at the end of this chapter in the Suggested Reading lists.) Even within the spinal cord and brain stem, 15 to 20 per cent of the fibers in each ascending pain pathway either go to the thalamic nuclei for the other pathway or interconnect with the other path somewhere along its route. No doubt still more complexity will be discovered in the future.

With such an array of ascending and descending pathways interacting with each other, it is easy to understand that sensory input regarding pain can be greatly modified. The nervous system used to be thought of as hard-wired and rigid. In fact, the reverse is true. Structural changes occur when we learn new ideas, enhancing transmission along preferred channels. Changes occur in interneuronal connections and synaptic density when new experiences occur (Chaplin, 1989). Neuronal plasticity is the basis of learning. Development of chronic pain is a learning experience, and people in pain need to learn how to control pain by "unlearning" the old lessons. Although the pain itself will usually persist, the suffering and disability can be greatly reduced by effective therapy at an early stage.

ANATOMIC BASIS OF PAIN CONTROL

Opiates (e.g., morphine, codeine) are temporarily successful in pain relief because there are opiate receptors in the central nervous system. Neurons whose function it is to turn the pain down once the brain has been alerted to a pain-causing situation release enkephalins or endorphins (endogenous morphine) within the brain stem and spinal cord in order to block continued transmission of pain signals (Bausbam and Fields, 1978). They do so by locking onto these same opiate

---

[3]There is some evidence that yet a third group of pain fibers ascend in the *dorsal columns* of the spinal cord to the nucleus gracilis (lower limb pain) and nucleus cuneatus (upper limb pain), intermixed with touch (Willis, 1985, pp. 202–205). At these nuclei, reception of pain information can be modified by higher centers. However, DeBroucker et al. (1990, p. 1230) quite emphatically deny this as a possibility in humans. There is also described a *spinomescencephalic tract* traveling with the spinotectal tract to the periaqueductal gray matter and superior colliculus in the midbrain (Wall and Melzack, 1994, p. 120; Willis, 1985, pp. 194–197). There is no universal agreement as to whether in humans such a pathway is a distinctly separate entity or whether it is just a collection of collateral branches to these midbrain areas from the spinothalamic tract.

receptors. Other substances released that inhibit pain sensitivity include serotonin and noradrenaline. Patients given opioids may say "I still feel the pain but it doesn't bother me anymore." In a very real sense this is the goal of chronic pain management. The pain may never be abolished, but, by stimulating the appropriate central nervous system pathways through cognitive-behavioral therapy, the pain will not be such a constant cause of concern. Stimulating these pathways is in the long run more effective than giving medications. The more exogenous opioid is given, the less will be produced endogenously. It is a losing situation. Restoration of the normal pain relief mechanism should be the goal.

Normally, ascending pathways for pain trigger a descending pain inhibitory response mediated by endorphins and related substances. The *raphespinal pathway*, with input from the periaqueductal gray matter, and the *reticulospinal pathway* from the nucleus raphe magnus and nucleus reticularis magnocellularis are two inhibitory pathways descending from the brain stem that terminate at the beginning of the ascending pain pathways in the dorsal horn of the spinal cord (Fig. 6–3). These are part of two powerful feedback loops designed to reduce sensitivity to pain. These descending pathways are influenced by inputs from the limbic lobe, that area of the cerebral cortex concerned with emotion. Through this mechanism, pain intensity may be increased or decreased. Cognitive-behavioral therapy to change attitudes and adjust goals and expectations works through these pathways.

The gate control theory proposed by Melzack and Wall (1965) makes it possible to understand how peripherally applied modalities, including acupuncture, might influence the nociceptive input at the spinal cord level. Nonpainful stimuli conveyed by large-diameter peripheral nerve fibers reduce the sensitivity of ascending pain pathways to incoming pain sensation (Fig. 6–4). Thus massage, manipulation, vibration, tactile, and other stimuli can reduce pain (Charman, 1989). There is also some evidence to suggest that, in addition to a similar effect on the dorsal horn cells, acupuncture can cause the periaqueductal gray matter in the brain stem to release endorphins.

Pain management must begin early. The management of pain, a central nervous system phenomenon, is similar in this respect to the management of connective tissue damage seen in muscles and tendons. The early response to connective tissue trauma is inflammation, and this is relatively easy to control. The later response is scar tissue formation, a much more difficult problem. The early neurologic response to a noxious stimulus is pain perception. If this is allowed to continue, secondary changes occur in the spinal cord and peripheral nerves that can give rise to allodynia, and even possibly reflex sympathetic dystrophy (Perl, 1994). The management of these complica-

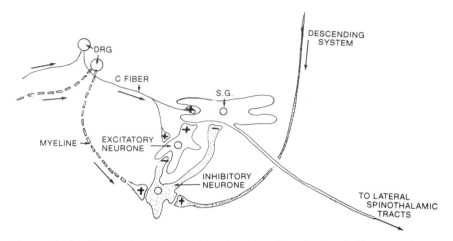

Figure 6–4. The pain gate. Nociceptive impulses in the C fiber are shown arriving at the beginning of the lateral spinothalamic tract, but ongoing transmission is inhibited by myelinated fiber and by the descending system. DRG = dorsal root ganglion. (Reprinted by permission from Cailliet R: Pain: Mechanisms and Management. Philadelphia, FA Davis, 1993.)

tions of long-term (persistent) pain is difficult, and the prognosis is poor.

UNDERSTANDING THE COMPLEXITY OF PAIN

Melzack and Casey (1968) suggested that there are three components of pain. The *sensory-discriminative* part of the pain experience is the result of spinothalamic transmission to the sensory cortex. The *cognitive-evaluative* component is the result of cortical assessment of the deeper meaning of this pain, with reference to ideas of significance stored in the association cortex and to memories stored in the temporal lobe (Fig. 6–1). For example, pain in the jaw from a tooth abscess may stimulate fewer pain fibers than an injection of anesthetic by a dentist. However, when the injection is given, knowing this is the dentist inflicting pain to prevent pain, and that the pain will be brief based on past experience, makes the dentist-induced pain easier to bear. Finally, there is the *affective-motivational* dimension to pain. The pain pathway projecting to the limbic lobe also receives input from past experiences. It is concerned with expectation of harm and desire to avoid it.

These aspects of the pain experience are now well accepted and have led to the development of effective pain control strategies. However, the principles on which they are based are by no means exclusive to pain. In order to explain the complexity of pain, it may be helpful to consider an example based on auditory sensory input that demonstrates how information is processed in the brain.

> Imagine yourself sitting in the middle of a half-mile-long railway bridge looking down at the river 500 feet below. Because it is a single-track bridge, you would have to run one-quarter mile, being careful not to catch your foot between the railroad ties, to escape from any train that might come. Of course such an event is unlikely or you would not be there. In fact the train is not due for 30 minutes and you spend those 30 minutes enjoying the sunshine, oblivious to the passage of time. Suddenly you hear a melodious sound. This is the *sensory-discriminative* aspect of hearing. From the primary hearing cortex, an electrical signal passes to the association cortex for hearing, and this sound, by comparison with various signals there, is identified as a train whistle. Long before you can start to enjoy the beauty of the sound, many other parts of your cerebral cortex have been notified, and now bring to the conscious level what in your daydreaming state you had forgotten: your location, the depth below, and the distance to run. However, before even this information can reach a conscious level, you experience fear and begin to run. The *affective-motivational* aspect of hearing has started you moving before you had time to experience and enjoy its *cognitive-evaluative* component.

One could devise a similar scenario for vision. It makes a great difference to how we feel about a flashing red light on a police car if we have just been speeding, or are stranded in an isolated area because our car has broken down. The same three dimensions—sensory-discriminative, cognitive-evaluative, and affective-motivational—can be described for all stimuli. Sensation is not a simple reflection of outside reality. It is very much influenced by what is going on inside one's head. This concept applies even more to the perception of pain.

Therefore, with better understanding of pain, the old distinction between mind and body (psyche and soma) must be discarded. The psyche and soma are one. With rare exceptions, we should never say "The pain is in your head." Yet, if it did not exist in the mind, it would not be appreciated as pain. Because this is so, if pain persists for 3 to 6 months or more, it is probable that it will have harmful effects on cerebral function in a general way. Such effects include fatigue, depression, loss of sleep, loss of interest in sex, anxiety, irritability, anger, frustration, and family and marital difficulties, as well as pain felt in areas other than the one originally injured. This cluster of symptoms is referred to by some as chronic pain syndrome. It is an unconscious and unhelpful adaptation *normally produced by a normal mind* in response to long-term pain. Unfortunately, some people use the term "chronic pain syndrome" in a perjorative sense, and many other syndromes share similar signs of psychological and social dysfunction. Therefore, the term is better avoided as a diagnosis (Merskey and Bogduk, 1994, p. xiii). However, the physical basis of these functional changes must be recognized.

Psychological Issues

Psychological issues in patients with chronic pain have been clouded by the lack of agreement on diagnostic terminology. Words such as "hysteria," which everyone seems to understand, have been dropped from use by the American Psychiatric Association (1994) while still being used with reference to pain by the IASP (Merskey and Bogduk, 1994) and even by those who create the scientific literature (Mai, 1995). The issues remain, however, and they can be broadly discussed under the following headings: conscious exaggeration of symptoms, unconscious intensification of symptoms, and the general psychological effects of persistent pain. The psychological effects of long-term pain have been listed in the paragraph above and can be understood as cognitive and emotional maladaptions that lead to behavioral changes. More must be said about willful conscious exaggeration and innocent unconscious intensification of symptoms.

Malingering is a *conscious* exaggeration of symptoms following a mild injury, or deliberate fabrication of symptoms following apparent injury, that is motivated by desire to avoid work or obtain financial or other rewards. This is rarely seen in injured workers (Ireland, 1995), but with experience is easily detected through inappropriate response to physical assessment.

Symptom magnification is an *unconscious* intensification of symptoms that may develop, for example, if insufficient attention is paid to the original injury by the employer, spouse, other workers, the compensation system, or even the medical profession. Factors producing and enhancing symptom magnification are discussed in Chapter 17. There is then extension of the pain well beyond the confines of the injured structure, and, if numbness is present, it does not correspond with the area supplied by a particular nerve or spinal nerve root. This is not malingering because it is an unconscious process, and real suffering is involved.

This phenomenon can best be illustrated by the following case history of an athletic injury in a teenage patient seen by this author many years ago, because in her case there was clearly no motivation for secondary gain. Although the symptom magnified was not pain, she did have pain-related numbness.

> A 14-year-old girl was referred to a sports medicine clinic with patellofemoral pain syndrome. (In those days all such problems were

called chondromalacia patellae.) When she had gone to her family doctor, he had told her the pain was nothing and it would go away, but it did not. When she came back to him months later, he referred her to a specialist, who gave her the same answer: "Don't worry, there is nothing seriously wrong with your knee." "Then," she said "my whole leg went numb."

Examination at the sports medicine clinic confirmed the patellofemoral source of her pain and found complete numbness in the lower limb distal to the groin and buttock crease. Her physical problem could finally be labeled and a reasonably successful plan of treatment with ice, exercise, and coated aspirin offered. One problem remained: What could be done about what was then called hysterical numbness? To address this, she was told: "Your brain is smarter than those two doctors. Your brain knew there was something wrong with your knee. When the second doctor said there was nothing wrong with it, your brain decided to make the leg go numb so that they would then have to admit there really was something wrong. Now that you know I have found out why your knee hurts, and that I can make it better, your leg won't need to be numb anymore." Immediately she replied: "You know what? My leg isn't numb anymore!"

Such a scenario is common in injured workers. Denial of what is perceived to be a legitimate problem leads to more extensive pain (allodynia) and nonanatomic numbness. Empathy and explanation helps to promote resolution because these patients know that at least someone understands their problems.

Not every case is so easy to diagnose. The help of a pain psychologist/psychiatrist may be required to explore what psychic needs may be contributing to symptoms of, for example, a conversion disorder or other somatoform disorders (American Psychiatric Association, 1994, pp. 445–469). Discussion of these conditions and their diagnosis and management is well beyond the scope of this chapter, but Chapters 13 and 16 will be found to be helpful.

Peripheral Versus Central Pain

It is both practical and correct to think of pain as consisting of two components, peripheral and central, with one or the other predominating. With an acute injury, pain is generated peripherally and transmitted centrally, where pain modulation occurs (e.g., the dentist-induced pain referred to earlier). When the acute injury is healed, the pain is gone. Thus for acute injuries, we are concerned with determining the peripheral pathology and look for a cure.

When the injury state persists for a long enough time, structural changes occur within the central nervous system that will perpetuate the perception of pain even long after the peripheral problem has healed. If a treatable peripheral source of pain remains untreated, it will feed nociceptive information into the central nervous system, making control of central pain difficult. Therefore, when treating chronic pain, we must identify and eliminate where possible any remaining peripheral sources of pain, while identifying and treating the central component.

TREATMENT CONSIDERATIONS

The central neurologic response to continued pain is a maladaptation that is structural in nature. Although these changes are often referred to as functional changes, all function is based on structure. The more we study the nervous system, the more we learn about changes in synaptic fields and the development of new preferred pathways for transmission of electrical signals that form a memory of pain to be played in response to particular cues. Psychotherapy can be nothing more or less than the induction of beneficial structural change within the central nervous system. Fortunately such changes are possible, but they are more difficult to achieve if the problem has existed for too long.

Therapy may also be seriously compromised by the patient's pre-existing mindset. This may range from hostility toward an employer to fear of further injury and consequent loss of needed income. There may be a pre-existing neurosis or personality disorder. Anderson and Hines, 1994, p. 148 state that children who are physically or sexually abused, abandoned, emotionally neglected or raised by those who abuse alcohol or drugs are more vulnerable to chronic pain. These also are organic, structural problems. Our present-day understanding of pathways within the nervous system allows us to make no distinction between structure and function, between anatomy and physiology. Such distinctions have been devised in the past to divide the workload of academics and of therapists. However, the mind and body are one, and a holistic approach is essential if we are to have any degree of success at all in the management of pain.

Likewise, we must treat central and peripheral sources of pain at the same point in time. Pain signals from injured tissue reinforce pain memory in the same way that pain behavior does, and maladaptive attitudes prevent the success of physical therapy being realized.

Treatment of chronic pain begins the moment the injured person walks into the examining room. By going from doctor to doctor and therapist to therapist seeking a cure and not finding one, such people will usually have arrived at some or most of the following conclusions:

Help must come from outside themselves.
A cure must be found but no one can find it.

Doctors are generally stupid.
Doctors and therapists do not really care.

Such conclusions must be shown to be false (Tollison et al., 1994). It is best to start with the last of these, by listening carefully to everything the patient wants to say and recording most of it. This shows that someone cares and that this individual is important. It will also give great insight into the nature of the problems, the injured persons's self-image, the nature of the work, the cause of the injury, and the injured worker's feelings about the work and the injury.

By doing a thorough physical examination, the health care practitioner reinforces the "I care" message and also distinguishes between central and peripheral sources of pain so that both may be treated. For example, if there was a wrist injury and pain that subsequently also involved the shoulder, it would be essential to exclude the possibility of pathology in the shoulder before approaching the subject of symptom magnification. Diagnostic feedback must be given to the injured worker with confidence and authority, but it will only be accepted if given following an examination that is perceived by the worker to be complete (Mai, 1995, p. 107). Although ancillary investigations are rarely needed, a nerve conduction study in the presence of glove/stocking anesthesia may be useful to demonstrate "with science" that there is no damage to the nerves. This is therapeutic. The purpose of the test is not to investigate but to treat. Radiographs, computerized tomography scans, and magnetic resonance imaging may be used in this way also, provided physical treatment is not delayed (see also Chapter 12 in this regard).

At the conclusion of an extensive examination, it is possible to then deal with the first two misconceptions, indicating that help must be found within the patients themselves, through natural (i.e., endogenous) pain control mechanisms, and that although control of the pain may be achieved, cure is not a reasonable goal. Psychological assessment is then arranged if necessary, and appropriate therapy continued.

REFERENCES

American Psychiatric Association: Diagnostic and Statistical Manual of Mental Disorders, 4th ed. Washington, DC, American Psychiatric Association Press, 1994.

Anderson D, Hines R: Attachment and pain. In Grzesiak R. Ciccone D (eds): Psychological Vulnerability to Chronic Pain. New York, Springer-Verlag, 1994, pp. 137–152.

Bausbam A, Fields HL: Endogenous pain control mechanisms: Review and hypothesis. Ann Neurol 4:451–462, 1978.

Bessou P, Perl ER: Response of cutaneous sensory units with unmyelinated fibres to noxious stimuli. J Neurophysiol 32:1025, 1969.

Chahl LA, Szolcsanyi J, Lembeck F (eds): Antidromic Vasodilation and Neurogenic Inflammation, Budapest, Akademiai Kiado, 1984, pp 7–25, 119–140.

Chaplin ER, Chronic pain: A difficult problem. Occup Med State of the Art Rev 4:433–447, 1989.

Charman RA: Pain theory and physiotherapy. Physiotherapy 75:247–254, 1989.

Corey D: Pain: Learning to Live Without It, rev ed. Toronto, Macmillan Canada, 1993.

DeBroucker T, Cesaro P, Willer JC, et al: Diffuse noxious inhibitory controls in man. Brain 113:1223–1234, 1990.

Granström E: Biochemistry of prostaglandins, thromboxanes, and leukotrienes. In Bonica JJ, Lindbloom V, Iggo A (eds): Advances in Pain Research and Therapy, Vol 5. New York, Raven Press, 1983, pp 605–615.

Helme RD, Gibson S, Khalil Z: Neural pathways in chronic pain. Med J Aust 153:400–406, 1990.

Hylden JLK, Nahin RL, Traub RJ, et al: Expansion of receptive fields of spinal lamina projection neurons in rats with unilateral adjuvant-induced inflammation: The contribution of dorsal horn mechanisms. Pain 37:229–243, 1989.

Ireland DCR: Repetition strain injury: The Australian experience—1992 update. J Hand Surg 20A:S53–S60, 1995.

Mai FM: "Hysteria" in clinical neurology. Can J Neurol Sci 22:101–110, 1995.

Melzack R, Casey KL: Sensory, motivational and central control determinants of pain: A new conceptual model. In Kensholo D (ed): The Skin Senses. Springfield, IL, Charles C Thomas, 1968, p 427.

Melzack R, Wall PD: Pain mechanisms: A new theory. Science 150:971–979, 1965.

Merskey HM: Classification of chronic pain syndromes. Pain 34(Suppl 3): 215–225, 1986.

Merskey HM, Bogduk N: Classification of Chronic Pain. Seattle, International Association for the Study of Pain, 1994.

Morris D: The Culture of Pain. Berkeley, University of California Press, 1991.

Perl ER: A re-evaluation of mechanisms leading to sympathetically related pain. In Fields HL, Liebeskind JC (eds): Progress in Pain Research and Management, Vol 1. Seattle, IASP Press, 1994, pp 129–150.

Rosomoff HL: Do herniated discs produce pain? Clin J Pain 1:91–93, 1985.

Tollison D, Satterthwaite J, Tollison J (eds): Handbook of Pain Management, 2nd ed. Baltimore, Williams & Wilkins, 1994, p 105.

Wall PD, Jones M: Defeating Pain: The War Against a Silent Epidemic. New York, Plenum Press, 1991, p 34.

Wall PD, Melzack R: Textbook of Pain, 3rd ed. Edinburgh, Churchill Livingstone, 1994.

Willis WD: The Pain System: The Neural Basis of Nociceptive Transmission in the Mammalian Nervous System (Pain and Headache, Vol 8). Basel, Karger, 1985.

SUGGESTED READING: GENERAL

Bonica JJ: The Management of Pain. Philadelphia, Lea & Febiger, 1953.

Cailliet R: Pain: Mechanisms and Management. Philadelphia, FA Davis, 1993.

Corey D: Pain: Learning to Live Without It, rev ed. Toronto, MacMillan Canada, 1993.

Gamsa A: The role of psychological factors in chronic pain. Pain 57:5–29, 1994.

Helme RD, Gibson S, Khalil Z: Neural pathways in chronic pain. Med J Aust 153:400–406, 1990.

Terenius L: Opioid peptides, pain and stress. Prog Brain Res 92:375–383, 1992.

Wall PD, Jones M: Defeating Pain: The War Against a Silent Epidemic. New York, Plenum Press, 1991.

SUGGESTED READING: ADVANCED

Chahl LA, Szolcsanyi J, Lembeck F (eds): Antidromic Vasodilation and Neurogenic Inflammation. Budapest, Akademiai Kiado, 1984.

Duggan AW, Furmidge LJ: Probing the brain and spinal cord with neuropeptides in pathways related to pain and other functions. Front Neuroendocrinol 15:275–300, 1994.

Fields HL, Liebeskind JC (eds): Pharmacological Approaches to the Treatment of Chronic Pain: New Concepts and Critical Issues. Seattle, International Association for the Study of Pain, 1994.

Light AR, Jones SL, Shultz RC: The Initial Processing of Pain and its Descending Control: Spinal and Trigeminal Systems. Basel, Karger, 1992.

Price DD, Mae J, Mayer DJ: Central neural mechanisms of normal and abnormal pain states. In Fields HL, Liebeskind JC (eds): Progress in Pain Research and Management, Vol 1. Seattle, IASP Press, 1994, pp 61–84.

Richardson BP: Serotonin and nociception. Ann N Y Acad Sci 600:511–520, 1990.

Wall PD, Melzack R: Textbook of Pain, 3rd ed. Edinburgh, Churchill Livingstone, 1994.

7
When Experts Disagree

Brian Martin _____

Gabriele Bammer

What can you do when experts disagree? One doctor says the worker has a real injury, another says the pain is psychosomatic, and yet another says the worker is faking. Whom should one believe? More to the point, how does one decide whom to believe? This is an issue in the case of chronic musculoskeletal problems, where different experts have different explanations for what is happening. They cannot even agree on a name.

There are two main reasons for this. The first is that these problems present challenges for those who make diagnoses. They are not as obvious as a broken arm. Therefore, there are quite a number of possible explanations that could be entertained at first glance. The second reason for the diversity of explanations is that there are strong social interests involved—vested interests, some may say—which means that workers, doctors, employers, and others have something to gain by preferring one explanation over another. This does not necessarily mean that anyone is consciously biased; it simply means that there are benefits to be had by sincerely believing certain points of view.

When divergent explanations for a phenomenon exist—chronic musculoskeletal problems, in this case—it is common to hear the cry: "Give me the facts!" Surely it must be possible to dispassionately look at the evidence and decide which explanation is best. Unfortunately it is not that easy. "The facts" are never unambiguous, even in fields such as physics and molecular biology. Different scientists may disagree about what counts as a fact. There may be disagreement

101

about the methods used to investigate the phenomenon or the way findings are interpreted. When scientists agree, it is not because the evidence is unambiguous and overwhelming; instead, they say that the evidence is unambiguous and overwhelming because they agree! At least, this is the perspective adopted by some sociologists of science, who argue that scientific consensus is a social process involving persuasion, negotiation, and resolution of conflict (Albury, 1983; Barnes, 1974; Feyerabend, 1975; Latour and Woolgar, 1979). One of the factors in this social process is the influence of interest groups.

To delve into the controversies over chronic musculoskeletal problems, we start by listing the main explanations and outlining some of the main areas of dispute. Then we look at a range of different interest groups, from people with these disorders to government, and comment on how they tend to align themselves in support of various explanations. Finally, in light of this survey of interests and knowledge, we suggest a few simple procedures for assessing conflicting claims.

EXPLANATIONS FOR CHRONIC MUSCULOSKELETAL PROBLEMS

We list here six common explanations of chronic musculoskeletal problems (Bammer and Martin, 1988, 1992; Meekosha and Jakubowicz, 1986). Supporters of each explanation typically cite certain evidence in its favor, but each explanation has difficulty with some evidence that does not fit. The latter we list under the category "anomalies."

Organic Injury

Explanation: the body suffers a real injury, typically affecting muscles, nerves, and/or tendons, as a result of rapid, repetitive movements, less frequent but more forceful movements, static load, or some combination of these

Common names: chronic musculoskeletal injuries, repetition strain injuries (RSIs), occupational overuse disorders, cervicobrachial disorders, cumulative trauma disorders

Evidence cited in support: reproducibility of symptoms; link with characteristic activities; aggravation by continuing the activities; growing body of pathophysiologic evidence

Pain and disability: real and work related

Anomalies: objective signs may not be present; symptoms may vary in location or seriousness; problems may not go away with rest or other treatment

Typical advocates: workers with problems; sympathizers
Beneficiaries if this explanation is accepted: workers
Typical responses: rest; avoidance of activities causing pain; biome-
chanical and organizational modification of workplace
References: Cohen et al. (1992), Dennett and Fry (1988), Helme et al.
(1992), Quintner and Elvey (1991)

Malingering

Explanation: workers are faking pain and disability to avoid work or
obtain compensation
Common names: malingering, faking, goldbricking
Evidence cited in support: observations or indications of workers freely
doing things they say are impossible or highly painful; unwilling-
ness to return to modified work
Pain and disability: not present
Anomalies: objective signs in some cases; prevalence in the most com-
mitted workers; similar problems related to recreational activities
such as sports
Typical advocates: sceptical employers, co-worker and insurers
Beneficiaries if this explanation is accepted: insurers; employers
Typical responses: disbelief; loss of pay; refusal to provide compensa-
tion; dismissal
References: Ireland (1986); Scarf and Wilcox (1984)

Compensation Neurosis

Explanation: workers unconsciously develop symptoms in order to
obtain compensation, either monetary or psychological (increased
attention and concern), often after recovering from a real injury
Common name: compensation neurosis
Evidence cited in support: lack of objective signs; variability of symptoms; recovery after financial payout received
Pain and disability: experienced as real but not linked to organic injury
Anomalies: objective signs in some cases; similar problems related to
recreational activities such as sports; lack of recovery after financial
payout received; loss of pay and sympathy after reporting prob-
lems; lack of objective signs for psychosomatic origin; lack of effectiveness of therapy
Typical advocates: sceptical employers and insurers
Beneficiaries if this explanation is accepted: insurers; employers

Typical responses: disbelief; counseling or therapy[1]; refusal to provide compensation
Reference: Rush (1984)

Conversion Disorder

Explanation: workers develop psychosomatic symptoms in order to escape (convert) psychological problems; no injury is involved
Common name: conversion disorder
Evidence cited in support: lack of objective signs; variability of symptoms; pre-existing or concurrent psychological problems
Pain and disability: experienced as real but not linked to organic injury
Anomalies: objective signs in some cases; similar problems related to recreational activities such as sports; lack of objective signs for psychosomatic origin
Typical advocates: sceptical employers and insurers
Beneficiaries if this explanation is accepted: insurers; employers
Typical responses: disbelief; counseling or therapy[1]; refusal to provide compensation
Reference: Lucire (1986)

Normal Fatigue

Explanation: normal pain and discomfort from physical work is interpreted as injury
Common name: normal fatigue
Evidence cited in support: lack of objective signs; variability of symptoms; recovery after rest
Pain and disability: real but not caused by underlying injury
Anomalies: lack of recovery after rest
Typical advocates: sceptical employers and insurers
Beneficiaries if this explanation is accepted: insurers; employers
Typical responses: rest; ergonomic changes at work
Reference: Hadler (1986)

Social Iatrogenesis

Explanation: workers with normal pain are encouraged by doctors and others to become patients with pain; a widespread belief in the hazards of certain activities becomes a self-fulfilling prophecy

---

[1]Although counseling or therapy should be the response, in our experience the assessment that leads to this diagnosis is a medicolegal one and hence treatment is rarely offered.

Common names: social iatrogenesis; pain-patient model
Evidence cited in support: lack of objective signs; variability of symptoms; "epidemics" of cases at particular times and places with no connection to objective conditions of work
Pain and disability: real but not caused by any underlying injury
Anomalies: objective signs in some cases; similar problems related to recreational activities such as sports; lack of objective signs for psychosomatic origin
Typical advocates: sceptical employers and insurers
Beneficiaries if this explanation is accepted: insurers; employers
Typical responses: change in social attitudes to normal pain
References: Bell (1989), Spillane and Deves (1987)

Areas of Debate

The above descriptions inevitably simplify the information about, and the case for and against, each explanation. More detailed accounts and arguments are readily available. There is a close similarity between compensation neurosis and conversion disorder, each of which offers a psychological explanation for problems, and between normal fatigue and social iatrogenesis, which complement each other. Beyond this, it should be obvious that it is quite possible for different explanations to be correct but only to apply in certain circumstances. For example, proponents of the normal fatigue explanation usually accept that some relatively well-defined disorders such as carpal tunnel syndrome are real, attributing less specific problems to normal fatigue, and proponents of the organic injury explanation accept that a small percentage of people do fake symptoms. Finally, our assessments of the typical advocates and the usual beneficiaries are accurate at most in a rough sense.

Some of the main areas of debate are indicated by the evidence and anomalies listed for the six explanations. In many cases, one explanation's supportive evidence is another explanation's anomaly, and vice versa. Nothing surprising in this! What would be surprising would be for a single explanation to explain everything. In that case, there would be no controversy. Some of the main areas under dispute are as follows (Bammer and Martin, 1988):

Objective signs (e.g., swelling). Critics of the organic injury explanation often point out that, although workers have symptoms—they tell of pain and disability—many exhibit no objective signs of injury. However, lack of signs is not a definitive objection. Other physical problems, such as migraine headaches, are widely accepted as real and organic even when there are no signs. Intriguingly, there is a double standard here. What are the objective signs for compensation neurosis or for any of the other explanations?

Underlying pathology. Many critics of the organic injury explanation say that there is no evidence of underlying pathology. Some say permanent injury of muscles through overuse is impossible. However, one explanation for lack of evidence of pathology is simply that medical science has not yet developed the methods or insight to explain what is happening. In addition, there is now growing evidence for possible underlying pathology (see Chapter 3).

Reproducibility of symptoms. Critics of the organic injury explanation often say that symptoms do not make clinical sense. Again, this may simply mean that clinical science has not yet come up with an explanation but that one is possible. Critics sometimes also dismiss plausible explanations. For example, some critics cite development of pain in the "other arm"—the one not originally injured—as a symptom that does not make clinical sense. However, it is possible that this pain developed because the "other arm" was overused through avoiding use of the injured arm.

Effectiveness of treatments. Critics of the organic explanation say that, when an injury does not respond to rest, some other explanation is needed. This is hardly a definitive argument, especially considering that there is little evidence that any of the treatments recommended for compensation neurosis and the like are successful.

An "epidemic" of cases. There have been great surges in reported cases of chronic musculoskeletal problems at certain times and places. For example, the number of reported cases of "repetition strain injury" in Australia skyrocketed in the 1980s. The idea of an "epidemic" suggests contagion rather than work-induced injury. Those who say that most cases are due to organic injury argue that injuries have been occurring in workplaces around the world for decades, but only occasionally are the circumstances favorable for workers to report them. When employers are able to dismiss injured employees easily, workers are hardly likely to make complaints. Critics argue that media reporting on a burgeoning problem of injuries encourages workers with normal fatigue to imagine that they are injured, makes malingering more likely, and suggests potential physical symptoms to those with psychological problems. The disappearance of an epidemic is also cited as evidence for a nonorganic basis for the disorders, but, as we have shown elsewhere, this is not necessarily the case.

In each one of these areas of contention, there are arguments for and against each explanation, arguments that in many cases can be backed up with studies and by the testimony of experts. Going deeper into the issue may not resolve it, because the divergent viewpoints influence the selection and interpretation of evidence at every level. Most crucially, which experts should one believe?

EXPLANATIONS AS A FUNCTION OF INTERESTS AND KNOWLEDGE

Incentives and Objectivity

In assessing work-related chronic musculoskeletal problems, the stakes are high. Is the injury real, faked, or psychological? Is recovery more likely through rest, exercise, therapy, or scepticism? Is it a worse mistake to disbelieve someone who actually has a real injury or to believe someone who is faking? What is the impact of a diagnosis on other workers? What measures should be taken in the workplace to prevent further problems? The answers to these questions can affect the health and livelihood of workers, the economic viability of enterprises, and the sorts of tasks and technologies that are introduced.

Science does not provide a final answer to any of these questions. Because the stakes are high, there are also strong incentives to pursue certain types of explanations. A diagnosis of organic injury validates a worker's suffering but can be costly to an employer or insurance company. A diagnosis of conversion disorder tells workers the problems lie in life outside of work and reduces immediate costs to employers and insurance companies. It should not be surprising that different groups prefer different explanations.

There is no conspiracy here, and probably little cynicism. It is safe to presume that proponents of different explanations sincerely believe their points of view. It just happens that there is a convergence between interests and preferred explanations.

For example, a psychiatrist may know a lot about psychosomatic disorders. Some psychiatrists may see patients who seem *not* to have organic injuries, so a psychosomatic explanation seems plausible. Once this explanation is tentatively adopted, the psychiatrist is attuned to look for supporting evidence and examples and to find holes in other explanations. Then an insurance company enters the picture. The company asks this particular psychiatrist, who is the one with an explanation to suit the company's judgment—that the sudden upsurge of cases must be something other than real injuries—to testify on its behalf. The psychiatrist testifies in court and, by being an open advocate, develops an even greater commitment to the psychosomatic explanation. (It would be embarrassing to back down at this stage.) The greater visibility of the psychiatrist leads to more referrals, more invitations to give testimony, and so forth.

The same sort of process can apply to proponents of any explanation. No malice or dishonestly need be involved. People of good will can legitimately ally themselves with different camps. This process can continue as long as there is enough ambiguity to allow different explanations to seem plausible, enough power and money to encourage advocacy of particular explanations, or both. The important thing to note is that interest groups, such as insurance companies, can have an influence on people's alliances, even though all concerned believe they are being fair and objective.

Is there some way to be fair and objective, not just in intent but in reality? We think not, because there is no universal standard, and there are no ultimate facts to which to appeal—at least not in a controversial area such as that of chronic musculoskeletal problems. Every one of us is influenced by commitments, beliefs, social location, personal experiences, friendships, aspirations, and the like. We can carefully examine and assess our beliefs and commitments, but there is no way to make them totally free of social influences—nor, perhaps, would we want to.

Nevertheless, the fact that perfect objectivity is not possible does not mean that all explanations are equally valid. Far from it. It is certainly worthwhile to examine evidence and listen to arguments in order to make the best judgment possible in the circumstances, and in accordance with one's own values. It is also important—and this is our main point—*to take into account potential vested interests when assessing evidence and arguments.*

Interest Groups

With this context, we now list some of the main interest groups involved in the controversy over chronic musculoskeletal problems. In each case, we suggest the sorts of explanations they are likely to prefer, noting that there are always some people who diverge from any pattern.

THOSE AFFECTED

Workers who suffer pain and disability are likely to believe that it is real—it feels real, after all—and to prefer the explanation of organic injury. Nevertheless, some find that other explanations seem to "fit" better. They may see a relationship with problems outside work or may be convinced that they are suffering from normal fatigue consequent on an increase in a normal workload.

CO-WORKERS

The responses of co-workers to workers claiming to have chronic musculoskeletal injuries can vary enormously. Some, especially those who have experienced similar problems, believe that the injuries are real. Others, especially those who have never experienced any problems, may blame those affected for trying to get out of work. The attitudes of workers are likely to be influenced by attitudes of employers, trade unions, and doctors and by stories in the media.

TRADE UNIONS

In principle, trade unions might be expected to stand up for workers claiming that they have been injured at work, but this often does not happen. Trade union officials can be torn in different directions: by the claims, beliefs, and disbeliefs of workers, by doctors, and by their own negotiating relationship with employers. When trade unions take a strong stand about the significance of workers' claims, this can have a powerful legitimating effect.

EMPLOYERS

In the short term, employers have an interest in denying the existence of disputable claims and in saying that problems are not work related. This is especially the case when injured workers can be dissed and easily replaced. Therefore, employers are likely to favor explanations of malingering, psychological origin, normal fatigue, and social iatrogenesis. However, if the number of workers affected is large or if it is difficult to replace them, or if those affected are workers with whom employers have highly valued personal relationships, then the problem may be taken more seriously. Measures may be taken to prevent injuries, such as introducing "ergonomic" furniture and equipment, changing work organization, and alerting workers to hazards. Employers may also introduce measures to rehabilitate and support those already affected. If such measures reduce problems, then the employer comes out ahead in the long run, whatever the explanation.

INSURANCE COMPANIES

When a large number of new claims of injury appear, insurance companies are likely to investigate with a sceptical eye, especially when plausible alternative explanations are possible. By contesting the organic injury explanation, insurance companies resist an entire class of claims. In contrast, if the organic injury explanation becomes widely accepted, then it is easier for insurance companies to pass on costs to companies via higher premiums.

GOVERNMENTS

Governments often ally themselves with employers. In some cases they are the employers themselves, and in other cases they have strong interests in promoting investment and employment locally. However, governments are subject to pressure-group politics. If popular pressure increases, governments may take action. It is important to remember that governments are not unified. Different government officials and employees—politicians, policy advisers, health care practitioners—may have different views and different agendas.

DOCTORS

Doctors can be pulled in different directions. They are influenced by their patients, by their relationship with employers, by their training and attitudes, by other doctors, and by other factors. Most doctors are likely to support the dominant explanation—the medical orthodoxy—at any given time. Usually that has been that chronic musculoskeletal problems are not common and not a particular problem. However, sometimes claims of injury become more visible and the organic injury explanation becomes the standard one, as in Australia in the 1980s. In any case, it is always possible for a minority of doctors to take individual stands. Medical researchers have an interest in promoting their particular perspectives. Doctors in workers' health care centers are more likely to take the complaints of workers seriously. Those who work for or receive many referrals from employers are likely to be more sceptical of the organic injury explanation.

Because doctors have a great deal of credibility in our society, they are often sought out to defend particular positions. A doctor who is willing to take a stand against the current orthodoxy may be championed by other interest groups, as in the case of the psychiatrist mentioned earlier.

SOCIAL MOVEMENTS

When a considerable number of people join campaigns for a certain sort of change in society, this can be called a social movement. There are many types of social movements, including the feminist movement, the environmental movement, evangelical religions, and promoters of computerization. A key function of a social movement is to move an issue onto the social agenda—in other words, to make it seem of significance to many people, whether they support or oppose change. In short, a social movement turns something into a "social problem" (Mauss, 1975).

For most of the time and in most places, chronic musculoskeletal problems have not been on the social agenda. Sometimes, when the social circumstances are right, social action leads to these problems becoming more visible and being taken more seriously. Beginning in the late 1970s, a few doctors at workers' health care centers in Australia began to publicize the pain and disability they perceived among manual workers from repetitive movements and static load. The term "repetitive strain injuries" was adopted by some doctors who wrote about the problem. Several groups took up the issue: women's health groups, trade unions, and workers themselves. Then the media became interested and this triggered a massive increase in visibility and activity with respect to RSI. The issue went from being a silent occurrence perceived only by isolated individuals to a social problem recognized by most of the population. The groups pushing RSI into visibility were, for the most part, not formally coordinated, but their efforts pushed in the same direction and thus they can be called a social movement. In this case, the social movement led to recognition of a social problem (Bammer, 1990; Bammer and Martin, 1992). Obviously, this movement favored the organic injury explanation. Previously, other explanations were seldom necessary, because so few individuals tried to obtain official recognition for their injuries. The explicit formation of the alternative explanations occurred in response to the movement's success.

Summary

The perspectives of every group and individual are influenced by their interests—influenced, but not determined. The point is that, when listening to what someone says, it makes sense to think about whose interests are being served by their viewpoint.

JUDGING CLAIMS

Given the complexity of the issue and the influence of competing interests, how should one proceed in trying to make a decision? There is no magical solution that avoids all the difficulties. We offer here some pragmatic guidelines.

Seek out a range of alternative perspectives. Do not rely on a few authorities. Ask to hear the arguments and see the evidence. For example, suppose you hear or read about the organic injury explanation. Are any anomalies acknowledged? If so, how are they explained? Are any alternative explanations mentioned? If not, why not? Look for material on other explanations.

Access the arguments and evidence in the light of interest groups involved. That means giving more scrutiny to claims made by those with a vested interest. "More scrutiny" means an extra dose of scepticism, not automatic rejection. After all, the fact that someone has a vested interest does not necessarily mean that individual is wrong.

For example, suppose the normal fatigue explanation is being presented by a medical researcher. Ask who employs the researcher, who provides research grants, and who pays for trips to courts to give testimony. If there seems to be a vested interest involved, give the claims of this researcher extra scrutiny, and listen to what critics say about the researcher's findings.

Apply the same procedures to other issues, including methods of treatment and strategies for prevention. Who benefits?

Look at your own interests. If the influences on you are likely to sway you in a particular direction, you can make a special effort to hear the other side. This is a challenge, to say the least!

CONCLUSION

We started out by asking the question, "What can one do when experts disagree?" The answer is that one must make one's own decision. There is no ultimate expert who can be trusted. In making one's own decision, it is valuable to seek out a range of opinions, perspectives, and evidence and to examine them with a sceptical eye, with extra scepticism when vested interests are involved.

Listening to all sides and being sceptical does not mean having no opinion. It is quite compatible with taking a stand and arguing strongly for a particular viewpoint. The more people there are who genuinely decide for themselves, without kowtowing to conventional opinion or whomever is doling out money, the healthier the debate, and ultimately—we hope—the healthier workers will be.

REFERENCES

Albury R: The Politics of Objectivity. Geelong, Deakin University Press, 1983.

Bammer G: The epidemic is over . . . or is it? Australian Society 9(April):22–24, 1990.

Bammer G, Martin B: The arguments about RSI: An examination. Community Health Stud 12:348–358, 1988.

Bammer G, Martin B: Repetition strain injury in Australia: Medical knowledge, social movement, and de facto partisanship. Social Problems 39:219–237, 1992.

Barnes B: Scientific Knowledge and Sociological Theory. London, Routledge and Kegan Paul, 1974.

Bell DS: "Repetition strain injury": An iatrogenic epidemic of simulated injury. Med J Aust 151:280–284, 1989.

Cohen ML, Arroyo JF, Champion GD, et al: In search of the pathogenesis of refractory cervicobrachial pain syndrome: A deconstruction of the RSI phenomenon. Med J Aust 156:432–436, 1992.

Dennett X, Fry HJH: Overuse syndrome: A muscle biopsy study. Lancet i: 905–908, 1988.

Feyerabend P: Against Method. London, New Left Books, 1975.

Hadler NM: Industrial rheumatology: The Australian and New Zealand experiences with arm pain and backache in the workplace. Med J Aust 144: 191–195, 1986.

Helme RD, LeVasseur SA, Gibson SJ: RSI revised: Evidence for psychological and physiological differences from an age, sex and occupational matched control group. Aust N Z J Med 22:23–29, 1992.

Ireland DCR: Repetitive strain injury. Aust Fam Physician 15:415–418, 1986.

Latour B, Woolgar S: Laboratory Life: The Social Construction of Scientific Facts. Princeton, NJ, Princeton University Press, 1979.

Lucire Y: Neurosis in the workplace. Med J Aust 145:323–327, 1986.

Mauss AL: Social Problems as Social Movements. Philadelphia, JB Lippincott, 1975.

Meekosha H, Jakubowicz A: Women suffering RSI: The hidden relations of gender, the labour process and medicine. J Occup Health Safety Aust N Z 2:390–401, 1986.

Quintner J, Elvey R: The neurogenic hypothesis of RSI. In Bammer G (ed): Discussion Papers on the Pathology of Work-Related Neck and Upper Limb Disorders and the Implications for Diagnosis and Treatment (Working Paper 24). Canberra, National Centre for Epidemiology and Population Health, Australian National University, 1991.

Rush J: The overuse of tenosynovitis. Med J Aust 141:614–615, 1984.

Scarf GE, Wilcox D: Alleged work-related injuries. Med J Aust 141:765, 1984.

Spillane R, Deves L: RSI: Pain, pretense or patienthood? J Indust Rel 29:41–48, 1987.

DIAGNOSIS _____

8
Diagnostic Criteria

Determination as to whether physical injury can occur in the workplace through repetitive activity has been greatly hindered by the use of terms that have no generally agreed-on definition, by basing conclusions on symptoms only, by failure to recognize the role of psychological factors and social influences on the severity of pain, and by failure to make a precise and complete diagnosis in individual cases. Physical injuries to connective tissue in the upper limb have been called repetitive strain injuries in Canada, but to many in Australia this term means a complaint that has no physiologic basis (D. Ireland, 1994, personal communication). Such terms must be abandoned if we are to communicate and understand each other. The mere fact that we use the term "disorder" (e.g., cumulative trauma disorder) suggests that something is wrong but that we are not really sure what the pathology is. In some cases this may be true, and the term is then justified, but a carefully conducted physical examination will usually clarify the situation.

We must never base our conclusions on symptoms only, as many thereby flawed epidemiologic studies have done. To do so leaves open the possibility that psychological and social influences may be responsible for these symptoms in some cases. There is then no accurate assessment possible of the magnitude of the problem. Such studies may relate more to perceived injury than to injury itself. Unfortunately, most medical doctors are either untrained, too busy, or too disinterested to make a proper assessment of work-related injuries. Consequently, there are no workers' compensation statistics about chronic work-related musculoskeletal disorder (or repetitive strain injury, or cumulative trauma disorder, or occupational overuse syndrome, or occupational cervicobrachial disorder or whatever they may be called) that have any validity whatsoever.

If we are to assess work-related injuries, we must first diagnose the injury through synthesis of history and physical exam, and then determine whether it was work induced or caused in some other way. We must examine both the worker and the work. We cannot state that there is a work-related injury unless we have evidence of

A *specific* pathologic change
To an *identified* tissue
Subjected to *sufficient stress* at work
To produce *characteristic* symptoms
Verified by specific tests.

Although the causative stress responsible for the symptoms may include psychological as well as physical factors, the pathologic change must be clearly a physical one.

HISTORY

The history will elicit the chief complaint, its duration, and conditions that make it worse or better. Patients often give the part of their anatomy as the problem (e.g., "my back" or "my elbow") when asked what their problem is. When asked "What is wrong with that area?", they often look at the health care practitioner as though he or she should have known the problem was pain. Nevertheless, the anatomic location of the pain is itself an important clue to the problem. For example, pain in muscles of the neck or forearm is usually due to static muscle contraction, whereas pain in the wrist or shoulder is likely to be due to tendinitis. Table 8–1 lists common examples. Those in parentheses are unlikely to be work related. This table is in no way intended to be comprehensive, but rather highlights the more common problems.

Usually, injured workers date the *onset of symptoms* to the time when it was bad enough to mention, but an overuse injury starts almost imperceptibly with what at first may have been considered normal fatigue. If a tendon or muscle problem is work related, there should be a clear history of symptoms occurring first at work after performing a stressful job and disappearing with rest, then progressing to pain that lasts longer. From this insidious onset, the injury goes

TABLE 8–1. Most Likely Causes of Pain According to Location*

Pain Location	Cause if Pain Only	Cause if Pain and Numbness/Tingling
Neck	Fatigue from static posture	(Cervical disc disease)[†]
Scapula	As above, plus scapular friction	
Shoulder joint	Rotator cuff tendinitis	Injured muscles of the neck pressing on nerves
Chest or arms	Overuse myalgia	Either of the two above
Back or legs	Acute muscle injury Static posture fatigue	Lumbar disc disease Sciatica
Elbow/forearm	Tendinitis Overuse myalgia	Injured muscles of the neck pressing on nerves
Wrist/hand	Tendinitis	Carpal tunnel syndrome (Cervical disc disease)[†]

*Adapted by permission from Ranney DA: Pain at Work and What To Do About It. Waterloo, Canada, University of Waterloo Press, 1990.
[†]Parentheses indicate the condition is unlikely to be work related.

through stages of gradually increasing severity. Various authors have given systems for grading severity of such problems based on similar experiences with sports injuries. The very descriptive three-stage division of Browne and colleagues (1984) is quite useful in showing how insidiously these problems develop.

A simpler version (Table 8–2) allows the health care practitioner to very quickly assess severity by asking only a few simple questions:

"Does your pain (or in the beginning did the pain) subside within 2 hours of leaving work?" (= mild)
"Is it still present when you are on your way to work in the morning?" (= moderate)
"Is the pain always present (continual symptoms)?" (= severe)

The purpose here is not just to grade the severity but to establish whether there is a pattern of gradually increasing severity, character-

TABLE 8–2. Grading of Severity According to Symptom Duration

Stage 1	Symptoms at work, disappear within 2 hr of leaving (mild)
Stage 2	Still present when attempting to sleep, possibly delaying sleep
Stage 3	Present in the morning before beginning work (moderate)
Stage 4	Daily symptoms all day, but resolve on weekends.
Stage 5	Continual symptoms (severe)

Stage 1 is mild, 2 and 3 moderate, 4 and 5 severe.

istic of chronic overuse problems, because by definition they cannot start acutely.

Next, we must establish *what makes it worse*. To a great extent, this helps with the diagnosis by identifying the structure injured, but it also forms the basis of later disability assessment when the need to specify job restrictions arises. Pain in the shoulder, for example, if coming from the neck will be aggravated by neck movements; if coming from the shoulder joint proper, by glenohumeral movement; and if coming from the scapular area, by movements of the pectoral girdle. Each will be attributable to different and characteristic job stresses.

What makes it better could be rest or some form of physical or medical treatment. If rest from the job helps (e.g., there is some degree of recovery over the weekend or when on vacation), this helps to implicate work as the causative or chief causative factor. The degree of recovery at rest indicates the severity of the problem—mild, moderate, or severe—as noted above. If time away from work does not seem to help, several possibilities must be considered. The worker may be exaggerating his or her problem to impress the doctor, or is aggravating the problem with activities outside work such as sports, housework, or hobbies. Alternatively, the real cause of the problem might be found elsewhere.

If forms of treatment that usually help chronic musculoskeletal inflammation have been to some extent successful (e.g., ice, anti-inflammatory medications), the suspicion of a physical problem may be confirmed, and recommendations given to continue this therapy. This is always a worthy dictum: If the treatment is helping, continue it; if not, then the therapeutic approach should be from another direction. Enquiring as to what helps and what does not avoids the embarrassment of prescribing something that has already been tried and failed. Beyond all this, and most important, this kind of questioning gives patients an opportunity for input to their own treatment program. Letting patients contribute their own experience will help make them realize their own importance to the success of that treatment program. Too often people may be encouraged to play a somewhat passive role in their recovery process. The truth is they must work hard to recover.

PHYSICAL EXAMINATION

Physical examination uses a lot of four letter words: *look* first, for deformity, swelling, color change, and calluses; *feel* for areas of tenderness, swelling, lumps, temperature changes, dryness of skin, or sweating; *move* to assess first active and then passive joint motion, noticing the presence or absence of pain on movement; and *test* for pain on resisted motion, muscle power, sensation, and circulation. Specific clinical tests relevant to the diagnosis under consideration must always be included. Occasionally, blood tests (e.g., to exclude rheumatoid arthritis), radiographs, nerve conduction studies, and the like may be necessary. All tests have their share of false positives and false negatives. Clinical experience and sound judgment are required to weigh the relative value of various symptoms, physical signs, and laboratory data.

The examination must be thorough and systematic, examining in detail first the problem area. After this, any related area that may have contributing pathology, or even be the main site of injury, must be examined. For example, shoulder pain may be the primary symptom, and evidence of rotator cuff tendinitis may be found on examination. However, if there is also a cervical problem, one must determine whether neck movements are the source of referred or radicular pain and thereby responsible for some or most of the symptoms. Likewise, on diagnosing carpal tunnel syndrome, it is well to realize that neck pathology may be responsible for the numbness and tingling in the hand. Specific tests for cervical neuritis, neck radiographs, and nerve conduction tests are then essential. Details of examination technique are found in Chapters 9, 10, and 11.

Good record keeping, standardized repeatable assessment techniques, and reasonable speed are all important. Standardized forms are best for this purpose; sample forms are provided in the appendices.

DETERMINING WORK RELATEDNESS

Job Task Analysis

Task analysis of some sort will be necessary to establish a causal relationship. When diagnosing a particular case, such analysis of the cause cannot always be performed in as sophisticated a matter as one might like (see Chapter 4). Nevertheless, the health care practitioner at least must always obtain a description of the job by history. The injured worker can be asked to "show me what you do," while the health care practitioner watches to determine such things as joint postures and cycle time. The worker can also be asked about rate of repetitive movements, how many units are produced per hour, the force required, whether there is high pressure or friction at the site of injury, any static or awkward postures, and the length and frequency of break periods. Environmental factors (excess heat or cold), use of gloves, and vibrating tools are also important considerations. If there is any possibility of examining the work site itself, this should be done. This will not only help in establishing a causal relationship but will also give insight regarding job modification so that the worker may more quickly return to work.

Assessment of Nonwork Activities

Hobbies and other outside activities, previous injuries, osteoarthritis, and other nonwork conditions could render a person more susceptible to work-related injury with less repetitive activities. Possibly the job is not causally related at all. Certain conditions classified as overuse problems are seen in the general public without any relation to work. For example, carpal tunnel syndrome in a given individual may be job related, yet most people who have it either have few job-related stresses or none at all. Muscle and tendon strains are much more common in industry than carpal tunnel syndrome, but are they *caused by* the work activity in this individual? Ranney et al. (1995) found carpal tunnel syndrome to occur in 9 per cent of workers exposed to highly repetitive work, well beyond the 1 per cent reported in the general public. Clearly this type of work puts many people at risk. However, when dealing with a single individual presenting for diagnosis and treatment, we still must determine if that person's work or other activities contributed most to the development of the injury. This can only be done by some form of task analysis and simultaneous investigation of nonwork activities.

Evaluation of Individual Variability

If a particular problem occurs commonly on the job, why does it affect one individual and not the worker next to her/him? This raises the question of tissue tolerance. We are all different; some people are stronger and more resistant to a particular injury than others. When a particular model of running shoe is tested to see how long it will last, it is placed on a machine that bends the sole up and down until something starts to wear out. Knowing how many times these shoes must bend on running a mile tells the manufacturer how many miles someone can run in them before the shoes will break down. The shoes of this particular model are alike, and all these shoes, unless defective, will break down at almost the same point.

How long can the runner run before his or her foot breaks down? Unlike shoes, runners are all different. The same applies to workers on the job. A particular amount of stress will injure the average worker, but who is average? Some of us are much stronger than others, some are weaker. Some workers may be predisposed to injury in some way that at present is beyond our ability to understand. It may be that what we do when we are *not* working may make us more prone, or less prone, to injury on the job.

Beyond tissue tolerance is the matter of pain tolerance. Financial and motivational factors, personality characteristics, and societal expectations affect our level of pain perception. Some patients volunteer the information that, although the pain is severe enough to interfere with sleep, they "cannot afford to take time off work." At the other end of the scale is a big, strong 58-year-old construction worker who cries at the mention of a visit to the dentist. On routine examination of factory workers as part of a large research project (Ranney et al., 1995), many people had tender areas about which they had not complained. Subconsciously, pain recognition had been suppressed until systematic assessment of these asymptomatic areas brought it to light. Some of them had other more painful areas that had absorbed their attention. Variation in response to pain in different individuals is truly amazing. More is said about this, and the anatomic pathways involved, in Chapter 6.

CONCLUSION

The key to diagnosis is not the presence of pain or other symptoms, but noting whether the anatomic pattern of symptoms and their severity is reasonable for the area stressed by the job, and whether physical testing verifies that the stressed area has been injured. For example, gripping a tool firmly may cause chronic fatigue of wrist extensors. The pain will be vaguely localized to the forearm extensor region. On physical examination, the findings will be more anatomically precise. There will be tenderness of the extensor carpi radialis brevis muscle but not of the brachioradialis, because it is not a wrist extensor but an elbow flexor. If the reverse is true on palpation, the task analysis should show repeated and/or forceful elbow flexion, not repeated and/or forceful gripping. If there is a poor match between physical job stress, symptoms, and signs, the stresses may indeed be there but are probably more psychological than physical.

Psychological stresses are important also, and very real, but cannot be dealt with effectively unless recognized.

The next four chapters present a detailed methodology for diagnosing chronic physical injuries encountered in the workplace, and the final chapter in this section indicates how psychological influences may also be detected. The appendices contain useful assessment forms and a list of the minimum clinical criteria required to establish a provisional diagnosis on initial assessment.

REFERENCES

Browne CD, Nolan BM, Faithfull DK: Occupational repetition strain injuries: Guidelines for diagnosis and management. Med J Aust 140:329–332, 1984.

Ranney DA: Pain at Work and What To Do About It. Waterloo, Canada, University of Waterloo Press, 1990, p 17.

Ranney DA, Wells RP, Moore A: Upper limb musculoskeletal disorders in highly repetitive industries: Precise anatomical physical findings. Ergonomics 38:1408–1423, 1995.

9
Neck and Shoulder, Back and Buttock

One important biomechanical function of spinal musculature is to convert a flexible multisegmented structure into a rigid structure. Segmental relaxation allows selective movement. Contraction confers stability, and this is particularily essential if there is bone or ligament damage. Few injuries frighten a worker as much as those to the neck or back. Such fear seems justified when one considers that the bones, ligaments and muscles of the neck and back protect the spinal cord. The muscles are programmed to tighten whenever the subconscious mind senses that the spinal cord is at risk. Hence there is a close association between an "uptight" attitude and muscle spasm. Management of the painful neck or back begins with an understanding of the cause and a determination as to whether or not there is risk to neurologic structures. As Chapter 12 indicates regarding low back problems, extensive investigations are not usually warranted, and are generally contraindicated once the safety of the nervous system has been established. This is surprisingly easy to do on clinical examination.

NECK PAIN

Neck muscles are classified as intrinsic or extrinsic, with intrinsic ones being confined to the neck itself, whereas extrinsic ones (e.g., the upper fibers of the trapezius) are attached both to the neck and the upper limb. All attach to the neck vertebrae, skull, or both, and all are important in stabilizing the head while the gaze is fixed. In this way, they all may suffer fatigue if the head is kept immobile for any reason. The intrinsics have their origin as far down as the sixth or seventh thoracic vertebra. Therefore, examination of the neck must include the upper thorax. Many extrinsic neck muscles attach to the shoulder girdle and therefore suffer fatigue not only with static neck posture but also when reaching up or when the arms are held up, as when typing or performing any manipulative tasks with the hands. The term *"tension neck syndrome"* is descriptive of the cause but indicates nothing other than a fatigue-induced chronic neck muscle disorder. This is often referred to as a muscle "strain," but, until we know more about the precise pathology, a better term might be "overuse myalgia," wherein myalgia simply means muscle pain.

As part of the usual look/feel/move/test routine, it is essential to search for tenderness of the upper fibers of the trapezius, the rhomboid muscles, the levator scapulae, and the three scalenes. All but the scalenes attach to the scapula and are suspenders of the upper limb. Because the intrinsic cervical muscles lie deep to the elevators of the scapula, it is hard to palpate them in isolation. Nevertheless, in the upper thoracic area, a pattern often emerges of tenderness that is vertical and always close to the midline for intrinsic muscles (Fig. 9–1). The extrinsic neck muscles are more oblique, somewhat more lateral, and capable of being moved lateralward with scapular protraction. Obviously, there is much overlap (anatomically and therefore diagnostically) between the intrinsic and extrinsic neck muscles and, although it is psychologically satisfactory to be precise, the distinction between various neck muscles may often be of little practical consequence.

Of greater significance is tenderness of the anterior and middle scalene muscles that embrace the roots of the brachial plexus, because swelling of these muscles, compressing the nerve roots, can produce pain, tingling, and numbness in the upper limb (*cervical outlet syndrome*) (see Chapter 10).

Movements of the neck are painful and may be limited in range when neck muscles have been strained for any reason. Injury to muscle is characterized by pain on the side where there is tenderness on moving the head so as to stretch these muscles (i.e., pain that the head moves *away* from). In contrast, pain on the side the head moves toward (e.g., rotation or lateral flexion *toward* that side) suggests bone/joint pathology such as arthritis or facet joint contusion (commonly seen in whiplash).

Facet joint pain may also occur in the absence of contusion if injured muscles have been allowed to heal in a shortened position. This is

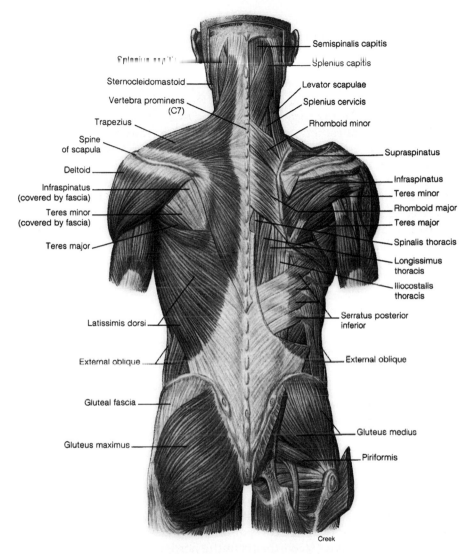

Figure 9–1. Intrinsic and extrinsic back neck muscles. (From van de Graaff KM, Fox SI: Concepts of Human Anatomy, 4th ed. Copyright © 1995 Wm. C. Brown Communications, Inc. Reprinted by permission of Times Mirror Higher Education Group, Inc., Dubuque, IA. All rights reserved.)

one reason why all muscle injuries should be treated by early mobilization. Articular cartilage is primarily nourished by synovial fluid, which enters and leaves the cartilage tissue through intermittent compression of the joint. In joints that are immobilized or, worse still, held under compression by tight muscles, cartilage degeneration results and pain endings in the adjacent joint capsule are sensitized. Pain on extension occurs, but there may be many reasons for pain on extension. A specific test for facet irritation is pain with extension plus rotation, provided the pain is felt in the facet joints on the side rotated *toward*. These facet joints must also be tender on palpation to justify calling the result a positive test.

To really prove the facet joints are the source of pain requires injection of local anesthetic into these joints under radiographic control and resultant temporary abolition of the pain (Merskey and Bogduk, 1984, pp. 108–109). However, a clinical diagnosis using the method outlined above will allow a treatment program to begin; if consequent muscle stretching gives relief, there is no need for any invasive procedure. Osteoarthritis of facet joints can also be a source of facet joint pain. This will be revealed on radiographs. Osteoarthritis pain is not usually relieved by traction or stretching exercises. What is true here of the neck applies equally well to the thoracic and lumbar areas.

SHOULDER PAIN

Shoulder Girdle Pain

Many writers have grouped shoulder girdle pain together with intrinsic and extrinsic cervical muscle strains and rotator cuff tendinitis under the heading "cervicobrachial disorders." When the prevalence of work-related injury is based on questionnaires only, it is not possible to subdivide this group. The more precisely we study mechanisms of injury, however, the more important it becomes to narrow the diagnosis down to specific structures as much as possible. This can only be done by physical examination (see Table 9–1). For example, degenerative osteoarthritis of the acromioclavicular joint gives shoulder pain that is aggravated by shoulder girdle movements, reaching forward or upward or both. One could argue whether the degeneration was the result of repetitive movement, but, because there are so many other etiologic factors involved in this condition, repetitive movement is neither a necessary nor a sufficient cause. A questionnaire response would falsely identify such a person as having a problem caused by repetitive work and a physical exam would not. Therefore, when examining the pectoral girdle (i.e., shoulder girdle) for the source of pain on shoulder movement, it is important to examine all parts. The examination should start with the sternoclavicular joint, clavicle, acromioclavicular joint, spine of the scapula,

TABLE 9–1. Differentiating Sources of Neck/Shoulder Pain

SOURCE	SITE OF PAIN	AUGMENTED BY	TENDERNESS
Cervical intrinsic muscles	Back or side of neck	Neck rotation, looking down, NOT by lifting	Neck/upper back, even down to T7 close to midline
Trapezius (upper fibers)	Top of shoulder; maybe neck also	Always lifting, extreme neck movements	Mastoid process to acromion, and all points medial to this
Subscapular (triction)	Scapular region	Scapular movement on chest wall	Rib angles 2–6
Rotator cuff tendons	Deltoid area (lateral arm)	Raising arm (not scapula)	Front of shoulder

muscles above and below it, and pectoral muscles and then concentrate on the adjacent rib angles, before moving on to the glenohumeral or shoulder joint proper.

Scapulothoracic Pain Syndrome

Scapulothoracic pain syndrome, alias subscapular bursitis, is the only shoulder girdle problem other than pectoral muscle strain that can be related to overuse at work with any degree of certainty. It is a common problem caused by rapidly repeated scapular movement, as when lifting small items from the side upward or by moving the arm horizontally. In these maneuvers, the medial border of the scapula rubs on the angles of ribs 2, 3, 4, 5, and/or 6. Tenderness localized to several of these angles is the hallmark of this condition. In severe cases, crepitation is felt on circumduction of the shoulder with the arm outstretched laterally. If such is present, manual compression of the scapula against the chest wall is usually painful and may increase the crepitation (Fig. 9–2).

If tenderness only is present, one must be certain it is confined to the ribs and does not occur between them. More generalized tenderness, if genuine, will probably be localized to the overlying rhomboid muscles and, if so, will move laterally with the scapula and be in a constant relationship to its medial border when the patient's hand is placed on the opposite shoulder.

Problems in the shoulder and arms are conveniently considered together because glenohumeral (shoulder) joint pain is characteristically referred to the deltoid region. It may also be reported as an anterior shoulder pain, and thus we must also remember to palpate for pectoral muscle tenderness.

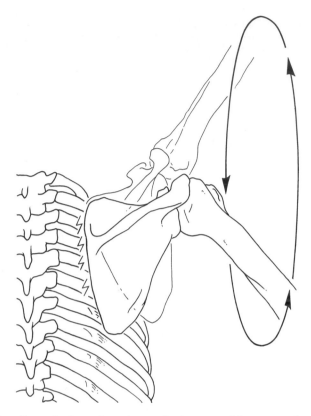

Figure 9–2. Scapulothoracic pain can be increased by manual compression of the scapula against rib angles 2 through 6 during arm circumduction.

Rotator Cuff Tendinitis

Rotator cuff tendinitis is frequently seen in individuals who work with their hands above their heads (e.g., painters) or with their arms horizontal. It may also be seen where work involves repetitive glenohumeral abduction, flexion, or both to or beyond 90 degrees. As a result of a prolonged static posture of flexion or abduction or repeated movement in these directions, the supraspinatus tendon becomes impinged on the coracoacromial arch and may thereby be damaged. The inflammatory reaction that results is primarily in the subacromial bursa (Uhtoff and Sarkar, 1991). Therefore, the alternative term "subacromial bursitis" is justified.

Identification of specific areas of tenderness is a simple matter if one observes that, on rotating the humerus (Fig. 9–3), the coracoid process does not move. Having identified this, the first mobile point to be noted on moving the palpating finger lateralward is the lesser

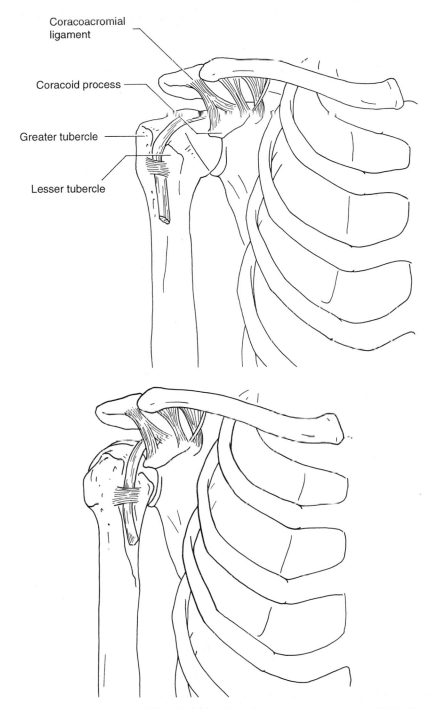

Coracoacromial
ligament

Coracoid process

Greater tubercle

Lesser tubercle

Figure 9–3. Anatomy of the shoulder. *Top,* Anterior view in neutral position reveals palpable bony points. *Bottom,* Internal rotation causes the tubercles to move but the coracoid process remains immobile. Having identified the coracoid process, the other bony landmarks can be identified with unmistakable accuracy.

tubercle. Superior to this, the sharp anterior edge of the coracoacromial ligament can easily be felt. Lateral to it lies the biceps tendon in its groove, and then, more lateral yet, the greater tubercle into which the supraspinatus tendon inserts.

The above description suggests that only the supraspinatus tendon is involved, and this is not the case. Although it is the most commonly affected, external rotation brings the subscapularis into contact with the coracoid process and internal rotation brings the infraspinatus tendon into contact with the acromion. Adjacent rotator cuff tendon inflammation is identified by noting specific tenderness at the sites of insertion of these tendons and by pain on resisted movements specific to their individual actions. For example, subscapular tendinitis is identified through tenderness of the lesser tubercle and pain on resisted internal rotation. Bicipital groove tenderness and pain on resisted biceps activity are characteristic of bicipital tendinitis. Supraspinatus and infraspinatus tendinitis will feature tenderness of the greater tubercle with pain on resisted abduction and external rotation, respectively. One should not be surprised to find widespread, more global, tenderness of the rotator cuff tendons, because the inflammation is rarely confined to one tendon.

Positive impingement tests (Figs. 9–4 and 9–5) confirm the diagnosis, distinguishing the tenderness noted anteriorly, laterally, or both from that resulting from deltoid muscle strain (which may coexist) (Hawkins and Kennedy, 1980; Neer and Welsh, 1977). However, these tests may be falsely positive if the pain-producing problem is osteoarthritis of, or injury to, the acromioclavicular joint. If so, pain noted on adducting the arm across the chest after flexing the shoulder 90 degrees will confirm that the acromioclavicular joint is involved. However, the most reliable differentiation is made by instilling 1 to 2 ml of xylocaine into the subacromial bursa or 0.5 ml into the acromioclavicular joint. When the pain is abolished, the site of injection must be the source of pain. Conversely, persisting pain indicates an alternative source. This is important in workers who may have, for example, rotator cuff tendinitis combined with trapezius overuse, with or without the addition of psychosocial factors intensifying the pain.

In other than mild cases, there is a painful arc of motion. This is measured by either abducting the arm or adducting it after it has been raised, and noting the number of degrees at which the pain begins and ends as it moves through the coronal plane (Fig. 9–6). Periodic quantification in this way is the best guide to progress. Often the patient may claim that "the shoulder is no better," but improvement can be proven by saying, for example, that 2 months ago there was pain on adducting from 135 to 45 degrees but now the painful arc of motion is only from 110 to 70 degrees.

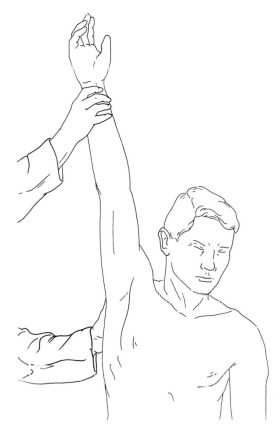

Figure 9–4. Impingement test of Neer. The arm is raised in the plane of the scapula.

Capsular Tears

Capsular tears can occur in one or more of several varieties, each of which can be identified on clinical grounds with reasonable certainty. An arthrogram, magnetic resonance imaging, or arthroscopy may subsequently be required to confirm the following clinical findings:

Small capsular tears are suggested by crepitation that is palpable subacromially with active circumduction of the shoulder, especially if the crepitation is coarse, is present also on passive shoulder movement, or both.

In the presence of a significant *tear of the supraspinatus tendon*, resistance to abduction cannot be maintained when the shoulder is flexed diagonally and internally rotated such that the thumb points

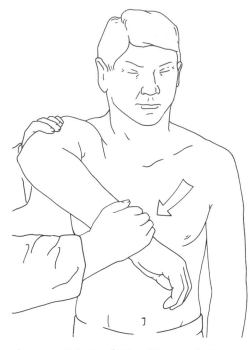

Figure 9–5. Impingement test of Hawkins and Kennedy. The shoulder, flexed 90 degrees, is rotated internally, causing the supraspinatus tendon to impinge close to the coracoid process.

to the floor. Reference to Figure 9–7 will indicate why this is also called the "empty can test."

A *subscapularis tear* may be suspected if the back of a hand placed on the small of the back cannot be lifted off it. To do so requires both extension and internal rotation together. Such a problem is unlikely to develop in the workplace, but rather suggests an acute, severe traumatic event.

Instability of the shoulder should not arise as a result of repetitive use but may be present from a fall or for other reasons, and may be seen as a noncompensable problem complicating a chronic work-related injury. Anterior instability can be assessed by abducting the externally rotated shoulder with one hand and attempting forward subluxation of the shoulder by pressing forward from behind the surgical neck of the humerus. Inferior instability can be assessed by a downward pull in the same area while the elbow is supported, using the Feagin test (Magee, 1992, p. 115). The examiner stands, facing the injured worker with the worker's elbow resting on the examiner's shoulder and pulls the head of the humerus downward.

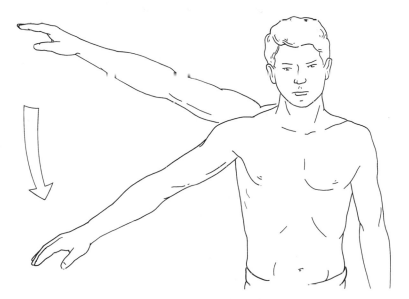

Figure 9–6. Painful arc of motion. As the arm is lowered in the coronal plane, a point is reached at which pain begins, and it continues as the arm is lowered further until a second critical point is reached and the pain disappears.

Posterior instability can be assessed by attempting to induce subluxation with a posterior thrust through the humerus when the shoulder is flexed 90 degrees.

Pericapsulitis

Pericapsulitis, or frozen shoulder, may occur as a result of an inflamed capsule becoming adherent to underlying bone. This is clearly evident when, with pain relief (e.g., injection of xylocaine subacromially), there is still a markedly limited range of motion. Typically there are three stages of frozen shoulder: (1) pain only, (2) pain and stiffness, and (3) stiffness only. Often a careful history in stage 2 or 3 will suggest the diagnosis.

Shoulder Girdle and Neck Injuries

Other shoulder girdle muscles to be palpated and stressed to determine whether they have been injured by repetitive use include the pectoral, deltoid, biceps, and triceps muscles. In addition, *the neck*

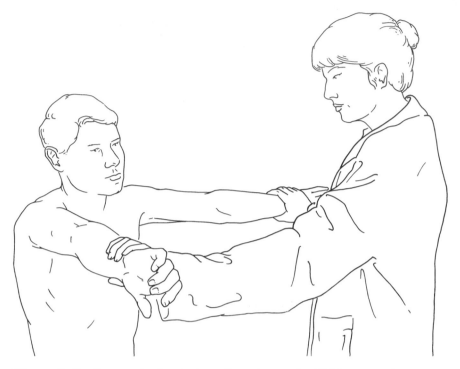

Figure 9–7. Supraspinatus test, or "empty can test." Downward pressure by the examiner is resisted by the patient. Because the arms are abducted in the plane of the scapula, resistance to downward pressure exerted by the hands of the examiner is offered by the supraspinatus muscle, and the position cannot be maintained if its tendon is significantly torn.

should always be assessed, if only briefly, with each shoulder complaint in order to exclude the possibility of shoulder pain originating in the neck. Although a great many alternative tests have been described (see Additional General References), the list of tests given on the shoulder examination form in Appendix III have been found by this author to be the most useful.

BACK AND BUTTOCK PAIN

As with the neck, back examination involves identification of tender structures by palpation, assessing range of motion, neurologic assessment, and performance of special tests. Schober's test is a means of reliably assessing back flexion that is recognized for its accuracy and found to be useful prognostically. This is discussed in Chapter 12 and illustrated in Figure 12–2.

Chronic Thoracolumbar Pain

Chronic thoracolumbar pain seen in the workplace may be caused by work or aggravated by it, may be acute or chronic in onset, and may be confined to the back or also radiate into one or both lower limbs. The most common diagnosis is the so-called *low back strain* precipitated by a sudden exertion that exceeds tissue tolerance. Table 9–2 compares this with other common conditions in a somewhat oversimplified way. The diagnosis is made on the history of a sudden application of force together with exclusion of the other conditions in this table. Unfortunately, there may be pain radiating into the limbs, causing concern that nerve root impingement has occurred. A good history will usually indicate its significance (see Leg Pain and Its Significance, p. 139).

In workers who have low back strain that is not resolving, when conflicts over compensation have occurred, *symptom magnification* may result. This features pain radiation (often below the knee) and numbness and tingling that follow a nonanatomic pattern. One confirmatory clinical test is the finding of a difference of more than 20 degrees when determining the point at which pain occurs on straight-leg raising when tested supine versus seated. Other signs of symptom

TABLE 9–2. Differentiating Features of Common Back Problems Resulting from Chronic Musculoskeletal Injury*

INJURY	CONDITION	CHARACTERISTICS
Muscle/ligament	"Back strain"	Extensive muscle tenderness Nonradiating back pain
Annulus of disc	Discogenic pain	Midline tenderness Pain relieved by extension
Facet joint	Facet joint syndrome	Tender beside midline Pain increased by extension
Sacroiliac joint	Sacroiliac syndrome	Tender sacroiliac joint Pain radiates to back of thigh
Nerve root	"Herniated disc"	As for discogenic pain Pain radiates below knee

*Serious problems that are quite uncommon are discussed in Chapter 12 under Assessing Red Flags. These consist of vertebral fractures, tumor, infection, and cauda equina syndrome.

magnification, such as flinching, jumping, or withdrawal when touched, use of a cane, or other pain behavior, may be seen.

The following sequence of movements may be very useful in distinguishing between symptom magnification and physical pathology:

1. With the patient supine, the straight leg is raised to the point of pain and lowered slightly until pain is relieved. Pushing the foot into dorsiflexion will then stretch the sciatic nerve, causing back pain that radiates down the limb if any roots of the sciatic nerves are irritable. If this causes pain (and only then), the examination should continue through the following three movements.

2. The knee should then be flexed 90 degrees and the hip brought slowly to 90 degrees of flexion. Pain on achieving this position is due either to hip or sacroiliac joint pathology, a severe disc prolapse, or symptom magnification.

3. Rotating the hip a little externally will not increase disc-related pain but will possibly increase pain resulting from hip or sacroiliac pathology. Hip pain is generally anterior, may be in the buttock, and is never midline in the lumbar region. In the absence of hip or sacroiliac pathology, pain on rotating the hip when flexed indicates symptom magnification.

4. Finally, placing the patient's foot on his or her opposite knee and allowing the flexed hip to abduct and rotate may cause back pain or increase it if there is sacroiliac joint pathology. This is Patrick's flexion-abduction-external rotation test of the sacroiliac joint. If midline pain in the lumbar region is increased or produced by these maneuvers, and other considerations exclude hip and sacroiliac pathology, there is now good evidence of symptom magnification. An empathetic discussion of the anxiety and the concerns these patients have, is the first step in chronic pain management.

Disc Injury

Disc injury may result in a tear of the annulus or a herniation of the disc nucleus through such a tear (also called a prolapsed disc). Although nerve root pressure caused by herniation of the nucleus of a disc is rare in the workplace, discogenic pain from the tearing of the annulus that precedes herniation is much less rare. In both cases, the tenderness is often confined to the midline at one or two levels and is generally much less extensive than in the more generalized muscle and ligament injury seen in a "back strain." Whatever the injury to the disc may be, unless there is an extrusion and sequestration of part of the nucleus outside the annulus, pain can be reduced by a program of back extension exercises. Extension causes nuclear material to move anteriorly just as flexion moves it posteriorly. Back extension exercises will aggravate facet joint pain; therefore, *the possibility of a facet injury should be excluded* in a manner similar to that described for cervical facet joint irritation.

Sacroiliac Syndrome

Sacroiliac syndrome consists of pain radiating down the back of the thigh from a sacroiliac joint that has been injured acutely or through repetitive trauma, and pathology in this joint often is unsuspected. The pain is always one sided, never central, differentiating it readily from discogenic pain. There is tenderness over the sacroiliac joint and there may be pain with standing on one leg or limitation of sacroiliac joint motion. Patrick's test for sacroiliac joint pathology is described above. Other tests for sacroiliac pathology have been described in the texts listed in the Additional General References at the end of this chapter.

Leg Pain and Its Significance

Many health care practitioners believe that a history of pain radiating into the lower limb from the back necessarily indicates pressure on a nerve. This is rarely the case, and it is often easy to distinguish nerve root (radicular) pain from referred pain in the lower limb even if the pain does seem to come from more centrally located structures. Irritation of the roots of the *femoral nerve* characteristically causes pain on the anterior or medial aspect of the thigh or both. Because the saphenous branch of the femoral nerve passes down the medial aspect of the leg as far as the ankle, the pain may extend this far. Irritation of *sciatic nerve* roots, or of the sciatic nerve itself (e.g., by an injured piriformis muscle), may give pain in the posterior thigh that usually extends below the knee posteriorly, laterally, and/or anteriorly, as shown in Figure 9–8. If there is numbness confined to the same dermatomal region, and increased pain on coughing, a clinical diagnosis of prolapsed intervertebral disc is justified. Associated muscle weakness may occur, but rarely, and this would constitute one of the few indications for referral to a surgeon.

Referred pain, in contrast, does not usually extend below the knee unless there is also symptom magnification, and then there may be related symptoms such as total-limb or stocking-type anesthesia. Referred pain in the limb is not usually as severe as the back pain and is generally an intermittent pain that occurs only when the back pain is more severe. In this respect, it may be thought of as an overflow phenomenon. The pain itself, like any associated numbness, may or

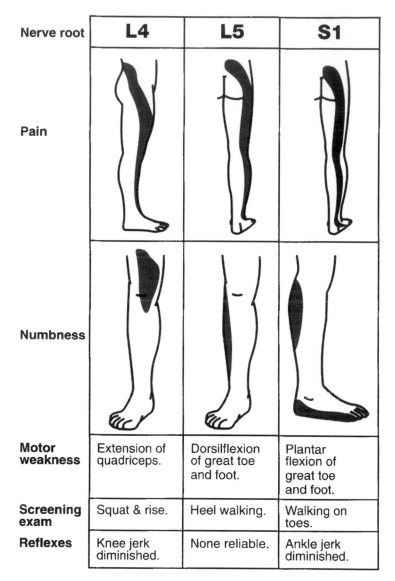

Nerve root	L4	L5	S1
Pain			
Numbness			
Motor weakness	Extension of quadriceps.	Dorsilflexion of great toe and foot.	Plantar flexion of great toe and foot.
Screening exam	Squat & rise.	Heel walking.	Walking on toes.
Reflexes	Knee jerk diminished.	None reliable.	Ankle jerk diminished.

Figure 9–8. Testing for lumbar nerve root compromise. (Reprinted from Bigos S, Bower O, Braen G, et al: Acute Low Back Problems in Adults: Clinical Practice Guideline, Quick Reference Guide Number 14. [Publication Number 95-0643]. Rockville, MD, Agency for Health Care Policy and Research, 1994.)

may not follow a dermatomal pattern. Coughing and sneezing may increase back pain, but, if it increases leg pain, this suggests that the increase in abdominal pressure is being transmitted to vertebral veins adjacent to nerves that are already experiencing pressure from a prolapsed disc. Referred pain is not increased by coughing or sneezing (see Table 9–3). Use of the words "usually" and "generally" in the above description of referred pain indicates there are no absolutes. Also, an injured worker may present with a mix of symptoms and signs that have features of both referred and radicular pain, but this is uncommon.

Other causes of chronic lower limb pain not related to the back must be mentioned because they may be found in a worker who has an injured back or an independent problem. They include vascular, traumatic, metabolic, and neoplastic conditions. Artherosclerosis deserves special mention. Anyone who complains of leg pain brought on by activity should have peripheral pulses examined to determine whether the cause could be intermittent claudication.

Fibromyalgia

Fibromyalgia deserves brief mention because, like osteoarthritis, it is a chronic musculoskeletal problem that may be found in an injured worker. It is not itself an injury, but a pre-existing fibromyalgia may be aggravated by a work injury, or even by work itself. It therefore needs to be kept in mind when examining a recently injured worker. Fibromyalgia also may appear for the first time weeks or months following an injury, and then the injury is assumed to be the precipitating factor. Not much is really known about this condition. It typifies the general rule in medicine that the less we know about a subject, the more is written about it. There have been many dis-

TABLE 9–3. Differentiating Referred Pain from Nerve Root Pain

CHARACTERISTICS	REFERRED PAIN	NERVE ROOT PAIN
Extent	Proximal to the knee	To and beyond the knee
Pattern*	May be nonanatomic	Nerve course or dermatome
Severity	Less severe than back pain	More severe or equal to back pain
Timing	When back pain worse	Independent of back pain
Cough impulse	No effect	Increases pain

*If numbness is present, the same pattern is found.

agreements about how fibromyalgia should be diagnosed and even whether it exists at all. However, a consensus has finally been reached regarding the features that characterize this problem.

In 1990, the American College of Rheumatology approved criteria to be met for the diagnosis of fibromyalgia. These are (1) that there should be a 3-month history of pain on both sides of the body, both above and below the waist and in the axial skeleton, and (2) that there should be tenderness at at least 11 of 18 specified tender points (Wolfe et al., 1990). The specified joints are listed in Table 9–4. These criteria received approval at the 2nd World Congress on Myofascial Pain and Fibromyalgia in 1992.

The pain is poorly circumscribed and aching in character, shifting from one area to another and varying in intensity on a day-to-day basis. Stiffness and fatigue are reported in 80 per cent of cases, sleep disturbance in 60 per cent, paresthesias of the extremities in 60 per cent, and headaches in 53 per cent. Other symptoms, such as anxiety and bowel disturbances, occur in less than 50 per cent of cases (Merskey and Bogduk, 1994, pp. 45–47). Fibromyalgia, myofascial pain syndrome, irritable bowel syndrome, and chronic fatigue syndrome have many features in common (Hadler, 1993). Much research is needed to clarify the distinction between them and the pathogenesis of each. Although there is a need to search for pathology, the constitutional, psychological, and sociological aspects also must be explored.

TABLE 9–4. Fibromyalgic Tender Points: Specific Sites*

Occiput	At the suboccipital muscle insertions
Low cervical	At the anterior aspects of the intertransverse spaces at C5–C7
Trapezius	At the midpoint of the upper border
Supraspinatus	At origins, above the scapula spine near the medial border
Second rib	Lateral to the second costochondral junction
Lateral epicondyle	2 cm distal to the epicondyles
Gluteal	In upper outer quadrants of buttocks in anterior fold of muscle
Greater trochanter	Posterior to the trochanteric prominence
Knee	At the medial fat pad proximal to the joint line

*Each of the sites listed may exhibit tenderness on one or both sides of the body. To confirm the diagnosis, 11 or more of the above 18 sites (each of the sites listed occurs bilaterally) must be tender. Digital palpation should be performed with an approximate force of 4 kg. Each tender point must feel painful on palpation, not just "tender."

REFERENCES

Hadler NM: Occupational Musculoskeletal Disorders. New York, Raven Press, 1992.

Hawkins RJ, Kennedy JC: Impingement syndrome in athletics. Am J Sports Med 8:151–163, 1980.

Magee DJ: Orthopedic Physical Assessment, 2nd ed. Philadelphia, WB Saunders, 1992.

Merskey H, Bogduk N: Classification of Chronic Pain. Seattle, International Association for the Study of Pain, 1994.

Neer CS, Welsh RP: The shoulder in sports. Orthop Clin North Am 8:583–591, 1977.

Uhtoff HK, Sarkar K: Classification and definition of tendinopathies. Clin Sports Med 10:707–720, 1991.

Wolfe F, Smythe HA, Yunus MB, et al: The American College of Rheumatology 1990 criteria for the classification of fibromyalgia: Report of the Multicenter Committee. Arthritis Rheum 33:160–172, 1990.

ADDITIONAL GENERAL REFERENCES

Many additional tests are described in the following books that may be helpful with respect to all parts of the musculoskeletal system.

Evans RC: Illustrated Essentials in Orthopedic Physical Assessment. St. Louis, Mosby-Year Book, 1994.

Hoppenfeld S: Physical Examination of the Spine and Extremities. New York, Appleton-Century-Crofts, 1976.

Magee DJ: Orthopedic Physical Assessment, 2nd ed. Philadelphia, WB Saunders, 1992.

SUGGESTED READING

Bigos S, Bower O, Braen G, et al: Acute Low Back Problems in Adults: Clinical Practice Guideline, Quick Reference Guide Number 14. (Publication Number 95-0643). Rockville, MD: Agency for Health Care Policy and Research, 1994.

Waddell G, Main C: Assessment of severity in low-back disorders. Spine, 9:204–208, 1984.

Waddell G, Main C, Morris EW, et al: Chronic low-back pain, psychologic distress, and illness behavior. Spine 9:209–213, 1984.

10
Elbow, Forearm, Wrist, and Hand

The extrinsic muscles of the hand lie in the forearm along with others that simply control the wrist. Some arise at or just proximal to the humeral epicondyles. At the wrist, these structures are represented by tendons, the transition occurring gradually in the middle third of the forearm (Fig. 10–1A). Examined in more detail, each of the forearm muscles that cross the elbow joint arises by means of a tendon that is usually very short. The superficial finger flexor has a much more complex architecture (Henry, 1959), but this need not concern us here. Those forearm muscles not crossing the elbow joint arise by fleshy fibers from forearm bones or interosseous membrane.

All these muscles insert into carpal, metacarpal, or phalangeal bones by means of long tendons that cross the wrist. Thus, the tenderness caused by pathology of muscle fibers or their attachment to bone or tendon will characteristically be located in the proximal two thirds of the forearm, around the elbow, or both. Characteristic features of conditions causing pain in the elbow and proximal forearm are summarized in Table 10–1. Tenderness at the wrist (if not caused by capsule or nerve inflammation) can only be due to tendinitis or tenosynovitis, because tendons are primarily what we find there. A notable exception is the flexor digitorum superficialis. Usually some of its fibers insert quite close to the wrist. Injury to these may produce a tender swelling just proximal to the wrist between the tendons of the flexor carpi ulnaris and palmaris longus (Fig. 10–1B).

145

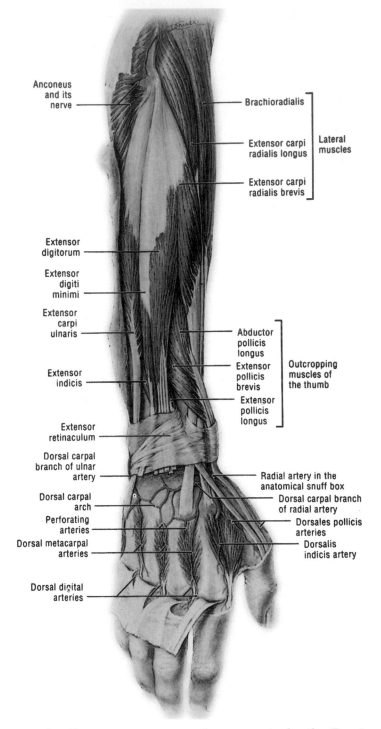

Anconeus and its nerve

Brachioradialis

Extensor carpi radialis longus

Extensor carpi radialis brevis

Lateral muscles

Extensor digitorum

Extensor digiti minimi

Extensor carpi ulnaris

Abductor pollicis longus

Extensor pollicis brevis

Outcropping muscles of the thumb

Extensor indicis

Extensor pollicis longus

Extensor retinaculum

Dorsal carpal branch of ulnar artery

Radial artery in the anatomical snuff box

Dorsal carpal arch

Dorsal carpal branch of radial artery

Perforating arteries

Dorsales pollicis arteries

Dorsal metacarpal arteries

Dorsalis indicis artery

Dorsal digital arteries

Figure 10–1A. Forearm extensor muscles: anatomic details. (Reprinted by permission from Moore KL: Clinically Oriented Anatomy. Baltimore, Williams & Wilkins, 1992.)

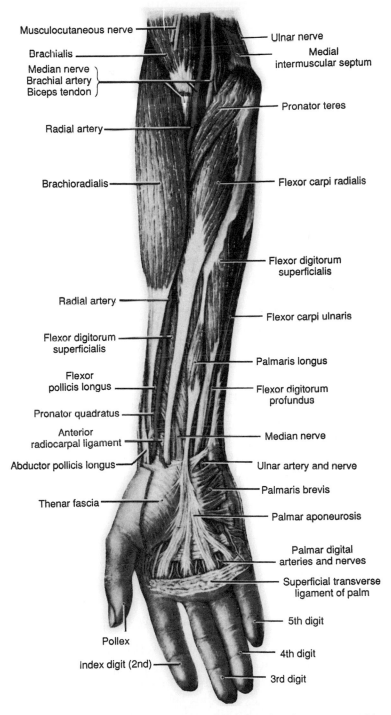

Figure 10–1B. Forearm flexor muscles: anatomic details. (Reprinted by permission from Moore KL: Clinically Oriented Anatomy. Baltimore, Williams & Wilkins, 1992.)

TABLE 10–1. Differentiating Causes of Pain in the Elbow/Upper Forearm

CAUSE	SITE OF PAIN	AUGMENTED BY	TENDERNESS
Triceps tendinitis	Back of elbow	Elbow movement	Triceps tendon
Arm myalgia	Above elbow	Elbow movement	Specific muscle
Synovitis	Elbow diffusely	Elbow movement	Each side of triceps tendon
Bursitis	Olecranon	Leaning on it	Palpable bursa
Epicondylitis/ tendinitis	Elbow: medial or lateral aspect	Forearm/wrist/ elbow movement	Epicondyle or within 1.5 cm of it
Forearm myalgia	Proximal forearm	Forearm/wrist/ elbow movement	> 1.5 cm from epicondyle over specific muscle

Terminology is important if we are to focus on pathology and its relationship to overuse activity at work. The term "tennis elbow," for example, has been used synonymously with lateral epicondylitis and tendinitis at the elbow. Sometimes these may be associated with radial bursitis or interosseous nerve entrapment. A purist would say that tennis elbow is an injury that only tennis players get, whereas those who look at mechanisms of injury would add that workers can get this same condition from similar types of activity on the job. However, if Joe Smith cannot work because he has tennis elbow, his employer might think that outside activity had more to do with causation than the job did. Those assessing and treating Smith must consider this possibility, but, after making a diagnosis of work-related injury, they should not send misleading signals to his employer.

Tennis elbow is a chronic strain of the wrist extensors in tennis players caused by repetitive high tensile loading of primarily the extensor carpi radialis brevis. Microtears in the tendon are associated with peritendinous inflammation that may extend proximally to involve the lateral epicondyle, deeply to inflame the underlying bursa, or more distally where muscle fibers arise along its course. There are often signs of collagen degeneration, and the tendon may be partially ruptured.

This pathology is also seen in workers whose wrist extensor mechanism has been similarly stressed, but then the term "extensor carpi radialis brevis tendinitis" is preferred. In such cases there may or may not be associated epicondylitis, but the tenderness does not usually extend more than 1 or 2 cm distal to the epicondyle. If it does, the muscle itself may be involved primarily or secondarily. If there is *no tenderness of the epicondyle or tendon* in its proximal 1 or 2 cm, there seems little justification in labeling the condition tendinitis. It is then quite unlikely that tendon-tearing high tensile forces are the cause. Such problems are more probably related to prolonged static activity, with the pathology being in the muscle itself, as discussed in Chapter 3. For this condition, the term "muscle strain" may be used, as it commonly is in the case of "trapezius strain." This is simply to indicate the site of some pathology that has been established clinically, not to indicate a physical disruption of muscle fibers. Some prefer the term "myofasciitis" when reporting forearm muscle pathology (Cohn et al., 1990). Because we do not really know in specific cases the precise pathology, the term "myalgia" may be preferred, as long as this is not taken to mean a psychogenic problem.

MUSCLE AND TENDON OVERUSE PAIN

Forearm muscle pain can be quite confusing. It is often overlooked or mislabled in spite of the fact that it is quite common (Pascarelli and Kella, 1993; Ranney et al., 1992, 1995). However, a sound knowledge of functional anatomy and a meticulous examination technique allow precise identification of the injured structures. The symptom of muscle pain may not always be well localized by the patient, but, when resisted activity produces pain in a muscle, its location will be correctly identified by the injured worker as being at what appears to be the muscle-tendon junction, and this will exactly correspond to the site of tenderness. Although injured tendons are less likely to be painful with resisted activity, they can be more precisely identified on palpation than can muscles, which tend to overlap each other.

The examination[1] should begin with palpation of the biceps and triceps if this has not been done previously. The lack of tenderness in muscles known not to be subjected to overuse helps legitimize the positive findings in those that are. The examiner can proceed from there to the lateral epicondyle, the extensor muscles, the medial epicondyle, and the flexor muscles in that order. The hand and wrist may be assessed as a unit after or before the forearm, thus concentrating on muscles at one point and tendons at another (see the assessment form in Appendix III). Which comes first is of little consequence and could depend on the stated location of the injured worker's pain.

---

[1]This discussion is reprinted, with modifications, by permission from Ranney DA: Work-related chronic injuries of the forearm and hand: Their specific diagnosis and management. Ergonomics 36:871–880, 1993.

Forearm Extensor Muscle Palpation

Identification of specific forearm extensor muscles is particularly easy (see Figs. 10–1A and 10–2). After palpating the lateral epicondyle, the examiner should follow distalward in the direction of the *third metacarpal* while rotating the forearm as the fingers pass across the rotating head of the radius just distal to the lateral epicondyle. They are now over the extensor carpi radialis brevis. This is the only pure wrist extensor. Its course can be traced to the midforearm and beyond, noting any tenderness. Similarly, the course of the extensor carpi radialis longus can be traced by palpation toward the *second metacarpal*, where it lies between the extensor carpi radialis brevis and the brachioradialis.

Moving back to the lateral epicondyle, the fingers should now shift slightly toward the olecranon to overlie the common finger extensor muscles and again palpate in a distalward direction toward the *third and fourth metacarpals*. The extensor carpi ulnaris and anconeus muscles lie even further toward the olecranon. The extensor carpi ulnaris can be followed distalward in the direction of the *fifth metacarpal*. Resisting wrist extension with the fingers allowed to drop into flexion, and then resisting finger extension while stabilizing the wrist by holding the hand in line with the forearm, will confirm any doubts as to whether the location of tenderness is in the wrist or finger extensors. It may well be in both. Mill's maneuver for tennis elbow therapy (Mills, 1928) applies a passive stretch by pronating the forearm, *flexing the wrist*, and then straightening the elbow. When testing to confirm either lateral epicondylitis, extensor carpi radialis brevis

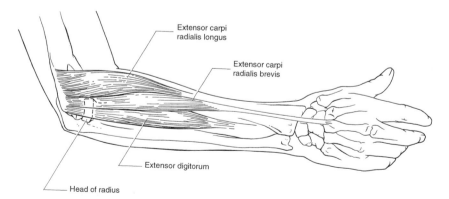

Figure 10–2. Identification of forearm extensors by palpation. The extensor carpi radialis brevis (ECRB) is shown arising from the lateral epicondyle of the humerus. The head of the radius can be felt rotating under its tendon when the forearm is rotated by the examiner. Other forearm muscles can then be identified in relation to this landmark (see text).

tendinitis, or wrist extensor muscle strain, I do a modification of this maneuver and straighten the elbow first, so that when, with the forearm pronated, flexing the wrist produces elbow pain, I know it is not due to elbow joint pathology.

Holding the forearm in the mid-prone position while resisting elbow flexion (Fig. 10–3) brings the brachioradialis into view. Palpation will now determine whether it was really this or the adjacent extensor carpi radialis longus that was tender. At the same time, one can easily locate the pronator teres (running from the medial epicondyle to the midpoint of the radius), and resisted pronation should be painful if this muscle has been significantly injured.

Forearm Flexor Muscle Palpation

Begin examining the forearm flexor muscles by palpating the medial epicondyle and common flexor muscle mass. Walk the fingers along the pronator teres to the midpoint of the radius, and then along each of the three wrist flexors distalward, in the same manner as was done for the extensors (see Figs. 10–1B and 10–3). Tenderness here indicates there is a muscle problem, but, because the forearm flexor muscles are arranged in three layers, palpation alone cannot identify the injured muscle. The examiner must rely on resisted movements of the wrist and fingers for precise identification. This is not a problem, because pain on resisted activity that is anatomically correctly localized legitimizes a complaint that otherwise might be in doubt

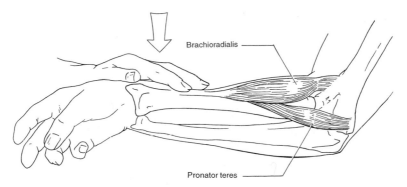

Figure 10–3. Identification of pronator teres. This muscle runs from the medial epicondyle of the humerus to the midpoint of the lateral aspect of the radius. Resistance applied to flexion when the arm is in the mid-prone position as shown makes both the pronator teres and brachioradialis taut and easily palpable (see text). Part of the supinator muscle (not shown) lies between them.

because (for other reasons) there may also be obvious symptom magnification.

An example of this is a patient who has forearm muscle injury that has been unrecognized. Anxiety has led to an exaggerated pain response. Now there is pain radiating up to the shoulder and glove-like anesthesia. Underlying these psychogenic symptoms is a physical problem whose recognition is the key to the entire clinical presentation. Workers who have been truly injured need correct treatment for the precise physical injury and also correction of the psychological and sociological problems that are responsible for symptom magnification, as discussed in later chapters.

With the forearm supine and resting on the table, thumb abduction induces contraction of the palmaris longus muscle (Fig. 10–4). Lateral to it lies the flexor carpi radialis (a radial deviator of the wrist), deep to which is the flexor of the thumb. Medial to the palmaris longus lies the flexor carpi ulnaris (an ulnar deviator of the wrist), and deep to both of these lie the superficial and deep flexor muscles of the fingers. The superficial flexor muscles can be easily identified, but whether pain on palpation emanates from them or from deeper flexor muscles can only be determined by looking for pain on resisted activity, under the guise of assessing strength.

Tendon Palpation

The extensor tendons for the wrist and digits are laid out in an orderly fashion at the wrist in six compartments (Fig. 10–5) and thus

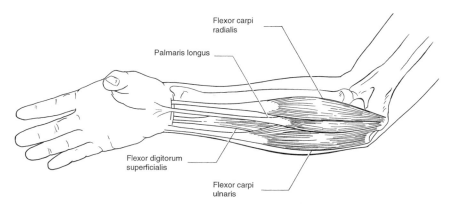

Figure 10–4. The palmaris longus tendon stands out with thumb abduction. This aids identification of the tendons of the other of two wrist flexor muscles at the wrist and of their muscle bellies in the proximal forearm. The superficial flexor tendons to the ring and middle fingers can be palpated between the flexor carpi ulnaris and palmaris longus.

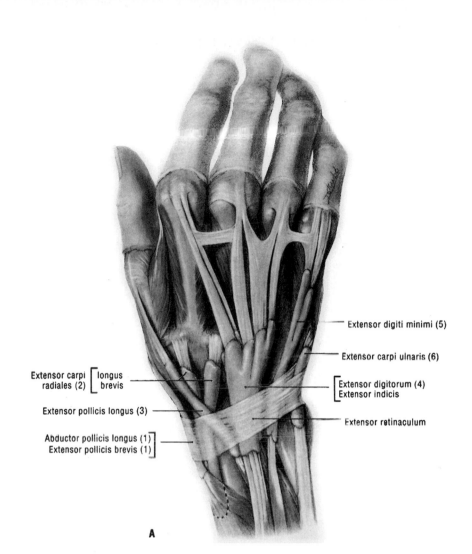

Extensor digiti minimi (5)

Extensor carpi ulnaris (6)

Extensor carpi radiales (2) [longus / brevis]

Extensor digitorum (4)
Extensor indicis

Extensor pollicis longus (3)

Extensor retinaculum

Abductor pollicis longus (1)
Extensor pollicis brevis (1)

A

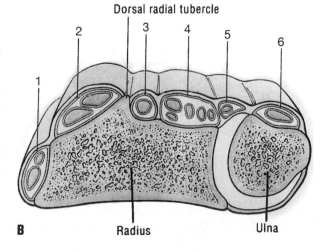

Dorsal radial tubercle

2   3   4   5   6

1

B

Radius   Ulna

Figure 10–5. Wrist extensor tendons: anatomic details. Numbers in Figure 10–5B refer to the tendons named in 10–5A. (Adapted by permission from Moore KL: Clinically Oriented Anatomy. Baltimore, Williams & Wilkins, 1992.)

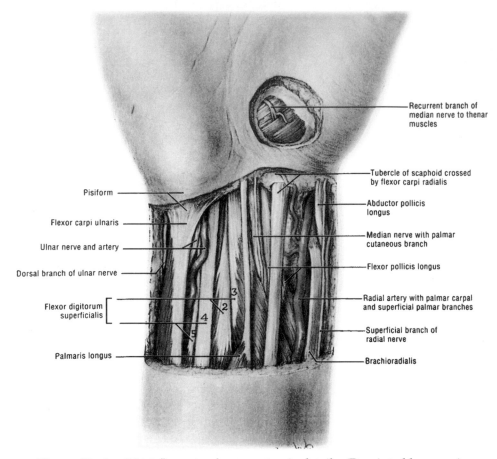

Recurrent branch of median nerve to thenar muscles

Tubercle of scaphoid crossed by flexor carpi radialis

Abductor pollicis longus

Median nerve with palmar cutaneous branch

Flexor pollicis longus

Radial artery with palmar carpal and superficial palmar branches

Superficial branch of radial nerve

Brachioradialis

Pisiform

Flexor carpi ulnaris

Ulnar nerve and artery

Dorsal branch of ulnar nerve

Flexor digitorum superficialis

Palmaris longus

Figure 10–6. Wrist flexor tendons: anatomic details. (Reprinted by permission from Moore KL: Clinically Oriented Anatomy. Baltimore, Williams & Wilkins, 1992.)

are easily identified by palpation. The wrist flexors are also easily palpated individually (Figs. 10–1B and 10–6). However, the digit flexor tendons, like their muscles, lie on a deeper plane. Therefore, only the tendons of the superficial flexors of the ring and middle fingers can be directly palpated. When looking for anterior wrist tenderness as a sign of tendinitis, however, it is well to remember that muscle fibers may insert into some of these tendons quite far distally. Swelling of flexor digitorum superficialis muscle fibers may produce a diffuse bulge that can be mistaken for a ganglion just proximal to the wrist creases and lateral to the flexor carpi ulnaris tendon. Also, the muscle belly of the pronator quadratus underlies the flexor tendons in the distal quarter of the forearm, and tenderness at this level could theoretically be muscular rather than tendinous in origin for this reason.

Pain on Stressing Muscles and Tendons

Resisted activity should be assessed after palpating the tendons. Then pain location under stress can be correlated with the site of tenderness and pain history. For example, resisted wrist extension should produce pain in wrist extensor muscles if these muscles have been injured and have been demonstrated to be tender. In cases of tendinitis (but only if it is severe), pain will be felt in the wrist extensor tendons where they lie on the dorsum of the wrist with resisted wrist extension, but in the finger extensor tendons (where they have been noted to be tender) with resisted finger extension (see Figs. 10–7 and 10–8). However, if pain is felt where the examiner's hand is resisting motion, unless this is itself a tender area, the patient's problem is at least in part psychogenic. Pain on resisted activity also must be localized to the structures that might reasonably have been under stress when performing the work alleged to be responsible.

Resisted thumb flexion (testing the flexor pollicis longus), flexion of all four fingers together (flexor digitorum profundus) and of each one separately at the proximal interphalangeal joint (flexor digitorum superficialis), followed by wrist flexion with relaxed fingers, allows one to test, in turn, the muscles of the three layers from deep to superficial (Figs. 10–9 through 10–12). If there is tenderness and also

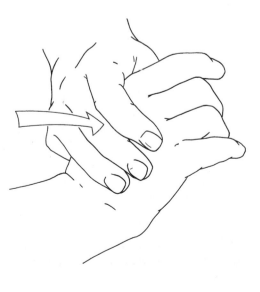

Figure 10–7. Resisted wrist extensor activity. With the forearm lying on a table, wrist extension is resisted manually and the site of any resultant pain identified. Note that the fingers must be relaxed. The examiner must be certain only the wrist extensors have been activated.

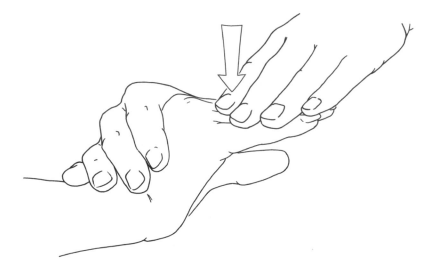

Figure 10–8. Resisted finger extensor activity. The wrist is supported in extension by the examiner's hand while finger extension is resisted with the other hand. As in Figure 10–7, the specific muscle tested must be isolated and the site of any resultant pain identified.

pain on resisted activity when the patient's attention is focused on the hand, this anatomic-functional correlation not only will identify the injured structure but also will affirm the genuineness of the complaint in those workers who have a legitimate injury. Others, seeking greater compensation and unaware of what tissue is being stressed, may complain of pain in inappropriate areas. Tests of legitimacy are summarized at the end of this chapter.

Tendons are capable of withstanding far more tensile stress before injury than are muscles, by a factor of 2:1 (Elliott, 1967). Although the level of force that an examiner can exert may be sufficient to produce pain in more severe cases, often it will not. However, to be completely confident in a diagnosis of tendinitis in those patients without pain on stress, the tenderness itself should be localized to tendons and not just spread diffusely around. If the tendon problem is not due so much to high tensile load, but rather is the result of friction caused by repetitive movement when under significant tensile load, one would not expect pain on resisted activity because the test, be definition, must allow no movement.

TENDON AND SYNOVIUM SWELLING

Where tendons run through tight sheaths, if they become swollen as a result of microtears, their excursion is painful. Swelling of the

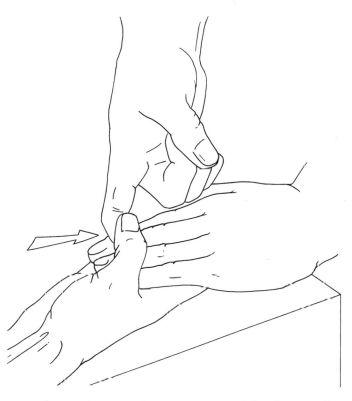

Figure 10–9. Resisted thumb flexion. Activity of the flexor pollicis longus is resisted in isolation, and any pain site identified. This should be along the front of the radius.

synovium lining the sheath and covering the tendon, swelling of the tendon itself, or both render the sheath too tight. The resultant increase in friction adds further damage. With time, the tendon becomes frayed, the frayed ends curl up to form rough areas, and crepitation can be felt. Although pain on stress may be lacking, letting the part go at the end of stress testing may give pain as the tendon under tension suddenly moves proximalward in its sheath.

In this regard, special mention must be made of the thumb extensors and long abductor. The short extensor and long abductor often lie together in one sheath (as in Fig. 10–5). However, there may be two or more sheaths. Whatever the number of sheaths, *de Quervain's tenosynovitis* is a common overuse injury. In the study by Ranney et al. (1995), it was more than half as common as carpal tunnel syndrome: 14 wrists versus 23, respectively. Finkelstein (1930) devised a test for this condition. With the thumb in the examiner's palm, the wrist is

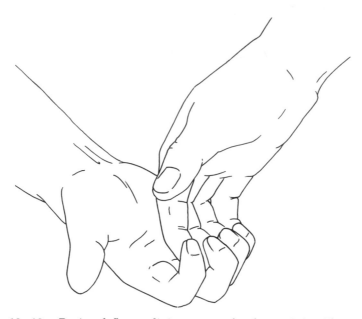

Figure 10–10. Resisted flexor digitorum profundus activity. Flexion of all fingers is resisted simultaneously, because the components to each finger tendon work together.

passively ulnar deviated. A positive test in the presence of tenderness of these tendons of the first dorsal compartment helps confirm the diagnosis, but, without sheath tenderness, it may mean nothing because this test can be mildly positive in normal people. Finkelstein's test will also be positive, but with tenderness being 2 to 3 inches (5 to 7 cm) proximal to the wrist, if the inflammation lies where the abductor pollicis longus and extensor pollicis brevis tendons cross the two radial wrist extensor tendons. This is referred to as *intersection syndrome*. In addition to tenderness, and possibly crepitation, there will usually be a boggy swelling resulting from enlargement of the intervening bursa, which lies deep to the muscle-tendon junction of the abductor pollicis longus.

INTRINSIC MUSCLE INJURY

The intrinsic muscles of the hand must be assessed for tenderness if there is a complaint of pain here. Resistance to activity of the finger intrinsics can best be provided if the patient flexes the metacarpophalangeal joints 90 degrees while keeping the interphalangeal joints straight. Significant muscle overuse will give pain on resistance as the examiner pushes against the volar surface of the proximal pha-

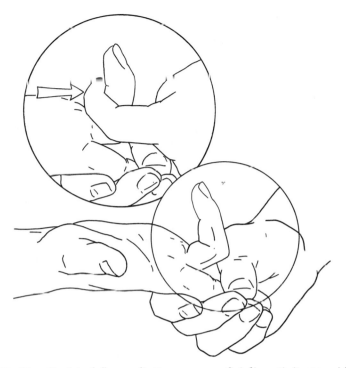

Figure 10–11. Resisted flexor digitorum superficialis activity to middle finger. This flexes the proximal interphalangeal joint. The other fingers must be held in hyperextension to overcome the effect of the flexor digitorum profundus. The ring and index fingers can be similarly tested, but because anatomic variations in the little finger are common, testing it leads only to confusion.

langes (Fig. 10–13). If the examiner applies his or her left hand to patient's left hand, and right to right, the index finger is always resisting the index finger, and so forth. This is also an excellent test of motor power (finger intrinsics are innervated by the first thoracic nerve and, except for the index and middle finger lumbricals, by the ulnar nerve). If pain is felt not in the muscle belly but in the tendon(s), between the metacarpal heads, intrinsic muscle tendinitis is thereby distinguished from joint ligament sprain.

TRIGGER DIGIT

Trigger digits may occur when there is a combination of high-force grip and high repetition, especially if there is local pressure over the sheath of a finger or thumb flexor tendon. Even pressure alone may be enough to cause this problem. For example, pressure over the the-

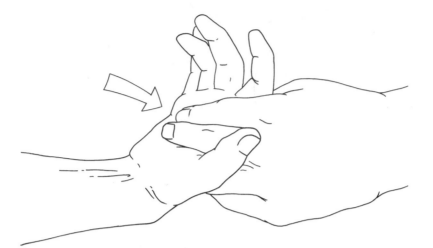

Figure 10–12. Resisted wrist flexor activity. Note that the fingers are relaxed.

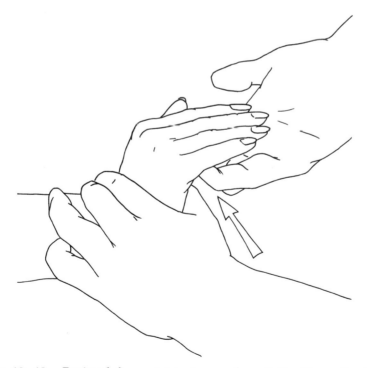

Figure 10–13. Resisted finger intrinsic muscle activity. The patient is attempting to flex the metacarpophalangeal joints against the resistance offered by the examiner's fingers. The examination should begin by asking that the interphalangeal joints of the fingers be kept straight.

nar eminence, as with gripping pliers or scissors, may produce flexor pollicis longus tenosynovitis. When a skin callosity is also noted at this site, it is hardly necessary to even obtain a job history (but it should be done as part of the routine). The symptoms may be snapping or catching. Tenderness will be noted at the entrance to the tendon sheath anterior to the metacarpal neck. If there is a history of snapping or catching but it cannot be demonstrated, it may be produced by pressure of the examiner's thumb at this point. In more advanced cases, a tender nodule will be palpable here. The production of this nodule and its location has been explained by Hueston and Wilson (1972) by comparing it to a thread being passed through the eye of a needle. The tendons are composed of spiraling fibers like those in a thread. When one strand is torn, it gets caught here and bunches up to form a ball that is too large to pass through.

JOINTS, LIGAMENTS, AND FASCIA

Confounding problems in the joints, ligaments, and fascia may mislead the unwary examiner; these include acute injuries and post-traumatic or chronic conditions. Acute problems include joint sprains and contusions. These, along with lingering post-traumatic problems (old fractures and previous soft tissue injuries), should be eliminated with the taking of an accurate history. Chronic joint pathology (e.g., osteoarthritis and rheumatoid arthritis) provides the main source of genuine confusion. Any pathologic condition may be aggravated by lesser degrees of overuse than would a normal joint. Although even a normal joint capsule may be stressed by repetitive motion, if these structures are tender and the tendons are not, the main problem is unlikely to be repetitive motion.

Rheumatoid Arthritis

Rheumatoid arthritis will classically present with other signs (e.g., synovitis) and multiple, often symmetrical, joint involvement. In the hand, the joints affected are usually the proximal interphalangeal joints (which assume a fusiform appearance) and the metacarpophalangeal joints, where there may be ulnar deviation as a result of loosening of the radial carpal ligaments caused by bone erosion. Before this disaster occurs, radiographs will show the erosions, allowing accurate diagnosis of rheumatoid arthritis and preventative synovectomy. Other diagnostic clues are the presence of subcutaneous rheumatoid nodules and an elevated serum rheumatoid factor.

Osteoarthritis

Osteoarthritis of the hand may present as painful deformities of the distal interphalangeal joints with dorsally situated lumps (Heberden's nodes). It commonly affects the thumb carpometacarpal joint. Tendons dorsal to this joint may appear to be tender because of work stress, but the real source of tenderness in such cases may be the underlying joint pathology. Tenderness on the joint's anterior surface together with pain on passive joint movement will suggest a diagnosis that a subsequent radiograph may confirm. The same principle applies to the wrist and finger joints.

We must bear in mind that osteoarthritis may itself be work related. Because it is so common, it is difficult to make a case for osteoarthritis resulting solely from overuse at work. However, in those who quite definitely have osteoarthritis and who have done the same repetitive tasks for many years, it is fair to ask how much the job may have contributed to these degenerative changes that in Europe have been given the alternative label "wear and tear" arthrosis.

Ligament Stress

Ligament stress may occur in any joint as a result of overuse—for example, in thumb carpometacarpal and thumb or index finger metacarpophalangeal joints from forceful repetitive pinching. Because this stress may be seen in otherwise normal joints, when seen in osteoarthritic patients, one must look into the work history to determine the role of overuse at work.

Dupuytren's Disease

Dupuytren's disease may be seen in the workplace simply because of its relatively high prevalence in white men after the age of 50 (Early, 1962). Metaplasia of the palmar fascia causes a nodule in and contracture of the palmar fascia, with resultant fixed flexion of the metacarpophalangeal or proximal interphalangeal joint. Although some authorities still consider this potentially related to repetitive trauma, most would agree there is no convincing evidence to support this view (McFarlane, 1991).

Kienböck's Disease

Kienböck's disease (avascular necrosis of the lunate bone) may be work related but often is not. When the ulna is short, the lunate is perched on the edge of the ulnar notch of the radius without the normal support of the head of the ulna (Fig. 10–14). In this situation (negative ulnar variance), normal forces transmitted from the palm to the forearm will traumatize the lunate. Similar trauma can occur if the ulna is too long (positive ulnar variance). However, when lunate trauma occurs without ulnar variance, one must suspect the external forces have been excessive. There may be a history of repeated direct blows to the front of the wrist or wrist ligament trauma.

When considering a diagnosis of finger extensor tendinitis, because the lunate lies deep to these tendons when the wrist is flexed, Kienböck's disease must be included in the differential diagnosis. Extending the little finger with the others flexed brings into prominence the extensor digiti minimi tendon where it crosses the dorsum of the distal radioulnar joint. Distal to this joint, deep to the extensor digiti minimi tendon and radialward, the lunate can be palpated by rolling the common extensor tendons toward the radial styloid process and flexing the wrist. Tenderness here warrants radiography, and, if the

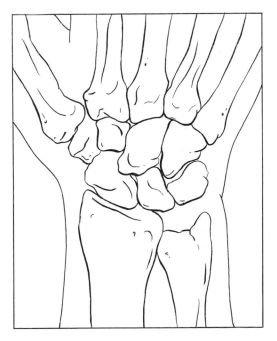

Figure 10–14. A short ulna (negative ulnar variance) leaving the lunate under pressure at the medial border of the distal end of the radius provides a predisposition for development of Kienböck's disease. When the ulna is of normal length, then the possibility of work relatedness should be considered (see text). (Redrawn by permission from Falconer DP, Donahue PJ, Barton ML, et al: Occupational hand fractures and dislocation. *In* Kasden ML (ed): Occupational Hand and Upper Extremity Injuries & Diseases. Philadelphia, Hanley and Belfus, 1991, p. 192.)

lunate is not collapsed or obviously fractured, a bone scan should be ordered to determine whether an unseen fracture is present.

Ganglions

Ganglions are never due to repetitive forceful movement over a long period of time but represent acute injuries, and the cyst-like swelling that results has usually been present a long time before it is brought to examination. In this sense only are ganglions chronic. Apart from those caused by mucinous degeneration of a tendon sheath, ganglions are herniations of joint synovium as a result of a sudden increase in bone-on-bone forces (e.g., with a heavy lift). They may or may not have been initiated at work but certainly will be aggravated by work. Most commonly they are on the dorsum of the hand, arising from the scapulolunate articulation. Always easy to diagnose when large, they initially may be so small as to be only a small tender swelling. Many times such an "occult dorsal wrist ganglion" is referred for diagnosis but, by the time the hand is examined, the ganglion has grown enough that the diagnosis is obvious.

Volar ganglions arise more deeply and from the radiocarpal or a variety of intercarpal joints toward the radial side of the hand. The stalk may be long and tortuous, giving rise to a ganglion at some distance from its joint of origin, or there may be no lump apparent at all. The cyst itself may only be found as a space-occupying lesion in, for example, the carpal tunnel when operating for carpal tunnel syndrome. When the diagnosis is in doubt, an arthrogram of the wrist may be used to show a connection (if any) between the wrist and the ganglion. In this case only, a positive result is helpful.

SYSTEM OF ASSESSMENT

A good system of assessment for the forearm and hand is as follows. After taking a good history, which includes a job history, palpation seeks to determine if there are tender structures at the site where pain is reported. Muscles, tendons, and other structures found to be tender are identified precisely wherever possible. Sensory assessment determines whether there is sensory loss to light touch and, if so, whether the pattern is that of a major nerve or nerve root or nonanatomic. Resisted activity is assessed after first saying, "Now I am going to test your strength" (which is done at the same time). If pain is apparent (without asking "Is this painful?"), the patient is asked where the pain is. Any special tests that may be indicated can follow. Range of motion assessment may be performed at the end or before testing for tenderness according to the examiner's preference.

TESTS OF LEGITIMACY FOR MUSCLE-TENDON PROBLEMS

Objective evidence of the severity of pain is unobtainable with currently available technology. However, an astute examiner, using the techniques described above, can be quite certain a muscle or tendon injury has occurred by stress testing based on three principles.

First, when stress is applied to a muscle-tendon unit, *pain experienced in an area already noted to be tender indicates pathology at that site.* This applies particularly well to forearm and wrist problems because of the complexity of the anatomy in this area (making it difficult for the patient to know the anatomy as well as the examiner does). However, there are several important considerations here:

1.   The application of stress must not be immediately after noting tenderness. This would allow someone with a large central component to the pain to anticipate the response and interpret tissue tension as pain.

2.   It is better to watch the face for signs of pain than to suggest there might be pain. Then, when pain is evident, the examiner can ask where it is.

3.   The patient should be told that muscle strength is being tested, which of course is being done at the same time.

4.   Tendons must be severely injured to be painful when stressed. Even injured muscles may not be painful when stressed, but, if a muscle is not, the degree of injury is at best mild, and the possibility of pain magnification or other centrally arising types of pain must be considered.

Second, *tenderness should be anatomically confined to tissues that might reasonably have been expected to be injured.* This test is applicable in a special way to tendons at the wrist that are not painful on stress. For example, tenderness of subcutaneous bone adjacent to a tender tendon indicates that it is not really the tendon that is tender, but rather the overlying skin. Examples are exposed areas of the radius (Fig. 10–5) and metacarpals. In such cases, in the absence of malingering, the tenderness is an area of secondary hyperalgesia or allodynia.

Third, when tissue is being stressed, *pain felt in another area usually indicates a false complaint.* However, one must be careful to position the upper limb properly so that other tissues are not stressed to con-

TABLE 10–2. Differentiating Severe Peripheral Versus Central Pain

STRUCTURE	PERIPHERAL PAIN	CENTRAL PAIN
Tendon	Tenderness *only* along the tendon	Adjacent areas are *also* tender
Muscles	Pain on stress testing felt *in* structure stressed	Pain on stress *incorrectly* localized
Both	Any pain on stress is in an area of tenderness	Dissociation of tenderness/stress pain
Nerves	Any sensory loss is anatomic (nerve/root)	Glove-like or patchy anesthesia
Skin	Nontender	Tender when pinched

trol posture. Finally, in some patients complaining of, for example, dorsal forearm pain, if this area is painful when wrist flexors are stressed, there remains the possibility that co-contracture of extensors when flexors are active may be the reason overuse of the extensors has occurred.

When soft tissue injury has been present for some time, the resulting *peripheral pain* may be increased by pain of central origin, as explained in Chapter 6. After healing has occurred, there may be just *central pain*, and until then the two may coexist. Both merit treatment, and in different ways. Whereas peripheral pain may be intermittent or constant, central pain is constant and usually described as burning in nature. Both will vary in intensity, but central pain tends to be more often severe, and the tenderness noted on palpation can be well beyond what one would see from even a severe acute soft tissue trauma. Table 10–2 indicates how these two very different sources of pain can be differentiated on examination when the pain level is intense.

REFERENCES

Cohn L. Lowry RM, Hart S: Overuse syndromes of the upper extremity in interpreters for the deaf. Orthopedics 13:207–209, 1990.

Early PF: Population studies in Dupuytren's contracture. J Bone Joint Surg 44B:602–613, 1962.

Elliott DH: The biomechanical properties of tendon in relation to muscular strength. Ann Phys Med 9:1–7, 1967.

Finkelstein H: Stenosing tendovaginitis at the radial styloid process. J Bone Joint Surg 12A:509–539, 1930.

Henry AK: Extensile Exposure, 2nd ed. Edinburgh, ES Livingstone, 1959, p 97.

Heuston JJ, Wilson WF: The aetiology of trigger finger explained on the basis of intratendinous architecture. Hand 4:257–260, 1972.

McFarlane RM: Dupuytren's disease: Relation to work and injury. J Hand Surg *16A*:775–779, 1991.

Mills GP: The treatment of tennis elbow. Br Med J *1*:12–13, 1982.

Pascarelli EF, Kella JJ: Soft tissue injuries related to use of computer keyboards: A clinical study of 53 severely injured persons. J Occup Med 35: 522–532, 1993.

Ranney DA, Wells RP, Moore A: Forearm muscle, strains: The forgotten work-related muscle disorder. Arbette Hälsa *17*:240–241, 1992.

Ranney D, Wells R, Moore A: Upper limb musculoskeletal disorders in highly repetitive industries: Precise anatomical physical findings. Ergonomics *38*:1408–1423, 1995.

11
Clinical Assessment of Nerves and Vessels

Nerve entrapment fascinates all those involved in the diagnosis and treatment of work-related injuries. Naturally, the most interested person of all is the worker, who not only has pain but also has numbness, tingling, or both as a source of anxiety and further discomfort. The primary nerve entrapment sites for the upper limb are listed in Table 11–1. Although the general prevalence is indicated, conditions that are generally uncommon may be quite common in specific industries where the risk factors for this particular problem are greater. A good example of this is vibration white finger, which occurs in workers exposed to high levels of vibration. This list is *by no means exhaustive* and merely serves, as does this whole chapter, to put into perspective the more common problems.

NECK AND SHOULDER

Cervical Outlet and Cervicoaxillary Syndromes

In the neck, nerve compression resulting from repetitive industrial overuse may occur through one of two different mechanisms. Carrying heavy loads on the shoulder may depress the shoulder suffi-

TABLE 11–1. Upper Limb Work-Related Neuropathies

CERVICAL
Brachial plexus neuritis (very rarely work-related)
  may affect any root of the brachial plexus
Thoracic outlet syndrome (rare)
  tends to affect the inferior trunk/lower roots of the plexus
Cervical disc herniation (very rare as a work-related problem)
Cervical osteoarthritis (very rare as a work-related problem)

SHOULDER/ARM
Lateral antebrachial cutaneous nerve compression (uncommon)
  musculocutaneous nerve passing through corachobrachialis
Saturday night paralysis (rare)
  radial nerve in spiral groove at midhumerus level

ELBOW/FOREARM
Cubital tunnel syndrome (uncommon)
  ulnar nerve between heads of extensor carpi ulnaris
Pronator syndrome (common)
  median nerve between heads of pronator teres
  median nerve between heads of flexor digitorum superficialis
Anterior interosseous nerve syndrome (rare)
Radial tunnel syndrome (uncommon)
Posterior interosseous nerve syndrome (rare)

WRIST/HAND
Carpal tunnel syndrome (very common)
  median nerve within carpal tunnel
Ulnar tunnel syndrome (uncommon)
  ulnar nerve within Guyon's canal
Wartenberg's syndrome (uncommon)
  superficial radial nerve deep to brachioradialis
Vibration white finger (generally uncommon)
Digital neuritis (uncommon)

---

ciently to compress between the clavicle and against the first rib (or apply traction to) the *first thoracic and eighth cervical roots*. This is a variety of thoracic outlet syndrome as currently defined. Pain with periodic numbness, tingling, or both along the course of the affected nerve root will be the presenting complaint. The relationship to overuse at work must be clearly established.

A second mechanism of injury would be compression of *any of the plexus roots* by swelling or fibrosis of injured anterior or middle scalene muscles or both between (or sometimes through) which these roots pass. Although much more common in acute injuries, such compression can occur as a chronic problem from static neck/shoulder postures or from reaching overhead, forward, or both in a variety of occupations. This is often referred to as a variety of thoracic outlet syndrome but often should be called *cervical* outlet syndrome (Ranney,

1996a). The subclavian artery and vein, together with the lower two roots of the brachial plexus, come *out of the thorax*. Clearly the *upper* brachial plexus roots do not, and it simply is not correct to call this type of problem thoracic outlet syndrome, but it is so classified at present.

Based on clinical tests that reproduced the patient's symptoms, a number of cervical nerve or neurovascular syndromes were described during the early part of this century. In 1956, Peet et al. suggested that "cervical rib syndrome, scalenus-anticus syndrome, subcoracoid-pectoralis minor syndrome, costoclavicular syndrome and first-thoracic-rib syndrome . . . be grouped together and referred to as thoracic-outlet syndrome" (p. 281). This was designed to reduce confusion, and it certainly has helped, but confusion still persists and more precise terminology is needed (Cuetter and Bartoszek, 1989). Because compression may not be at the real thoracic outlet (between the scalene muscles), but rather in more distal parts of what Anson (1966) called the cervicoaxillary canal, perhaps the term "cervicoaxillary syndrome" would be more helpful (Ranney, 1996a). Figure 11–1 shows these three sites.

The thoracic outlet is an opening between the anterior and middle scalene muscles. The inferior border of this opening is the first rib. It is over this first rib (or a cervical rib if present) that the subclavian artery and vein and the lower roots of the brachial plexus emerge from within the thorax. Unfortunately, leading authorities such as Travell and Simons (1983) and other writers (e.g., Mosley et al., 1991) define the thoracic outlet as the triangle formed by this rib and the *entire length* of the two scalene muscles. This area is in fact the scalene triangle. It is only the lower part of the scalene triangle that serves as a thoracic outlet. When there is a cervical rib or band, the seventh cervical root will also need to rise up and pass over the anomalous structure to reach the axilla, and may then be deemed to exit from the thorax. However, compression of roots C5 and C6 can never occur from below as a result of allowing the shoulders to drop, and should never be treated by strengthening shoulder girdle muscles (as suggested by Mosly et al., 1991, p. 362) or by resection of the first rib. If surgery is necessary, it should be a simple scalenotomy, done only if there remains a significant nerve dysfunction after scalene stretching exercises have been thoroughly performed. For this reason, it is essential to differentiate between cervical outlet syndrome and the other conditions currently grouped under the heading "thoracic outlet syndrome" (Table 11–2).

The *diagnosis* of thoracic outlet syndrome (as currently defined) is extremely difficult. Those with a high index of suspicion tend to overdiagnose this rare condition, and skeptical diagnosticians may miss it altogether unless there are symptoms of vascular compromise. The person affected will complain of painful tingling and possibly numb-

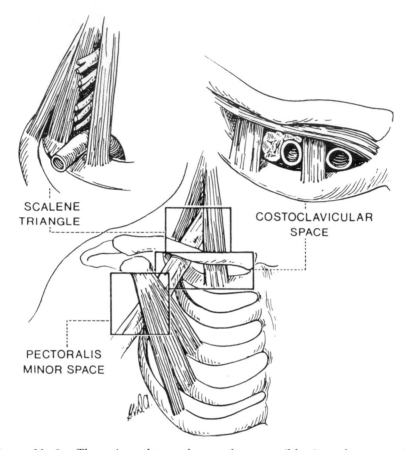

SCALENE
TRIANGLE

COSTOCLAVICULAR
SPACE

PECTORALIS
MINOR SPACE

Figure 11–1. Thoracic outlet syndrome: three possible sites of compression. (Reprinted by permission from Mosley LH, Kalafut RM, Levinson PD, et al: Cumulative trauma disorders and compression neuropathies of the upper extremities. *In* Kasdan ML (ed): Occupational Hand and Upper Extremity Injuries & Diseases. Philadelphia, Hanley & Belfus, 1991, pp 353–402.)

ness in the upper limb, which is usually present proximally and along the postaxial border. On examination, symptoms may be reproducible when the shoulder is abducted 90 degrees and externally rotated. There may be supraclavicular tenderness over the anterior and/or middle scalene muscle. This clinical picture is seen in most patients. These symptoms and signs are generally accepted as significant diagnostic criteria (Sanders and Haug, 1991, p. 4). Rarely will there be signs of overt nerve dysfunction or vascular problems. If there is any weakness, it primarily affects intrinsic *thumb* muscles. Because these are largely innervated by the median nerve, one might suspect carpal tunnel syndrome. However, sensory loss medially in the forearm

TABLE 11–2. Cervical Outlet and Cervicoaxillary Syndromes

ANATOMIC SITE	STRUCTURES AFFECTED	TESTS
"Cervical outlet" (new concept)	Upper cervical nerve roots	Modified Adson's ± 90 degrees abduction + external rotation
Thoracic outlet (redefined)	Lower roots ± subclavian *artery*	
Costoclavicular space	Any brachial plexus trunk ± subclavian *artery* and/or *vein*	Costoclavicular (shoulder brace)
Subcoracoid/ pectoralis minor	Any brachial plexus trunk ± subclavian *artery* and/or *vein*	Hyperabduction

combined with motor weakness laterally in the hand identifies this as a T1 nerve root lesion, of which thoracic outlet syndrome might be the cause.

Thoracic outlet syndrome is primarily a neurologic problem, but there may be arterial or venous compression, or both, as well. Based on symptomatology, thoracic outlet syndrome may be classified as neurogenic, arterial, or venous. Wilbourn (1988) introduced the term "disputed neurogenic" for the large subdivision of the neurogenic type in which objective diagnostic tests are normal. The *classic tests* for thoracic outlet syndrome may be useful, but there are many false positives and false negatives (Leffert, 1983). One should only consider a test positive and significant if it reproduces the patient's symptoms (Karas, 1990, p. 304). Simple obliteration of the pulse is not significant in a purely neurogenic case because this may be just a false positive result.

Adson's test (Adson, Coffey, 1927) involves deep inspiration, neck extension, and turning the head toward the examiner (Fig. 11–2). Many clinicians, including this author, believe that the test is more sensitive with the head turned away. As a quick screening test, this modified Adson test can be combined with manual costoclavicular compression and the Roos test: holding the shoulder in 90 degrees of abduction and full external rotation while palpating the radial artery (Fig. 11–3). The hyperabduction test (Roos and Owens, 1966), as seen in Figure 11–4, should also be performed, and if positive suggests the problem that Wright (1945) described in which brachial plexus components and subclavian vessels might be "stretched around and

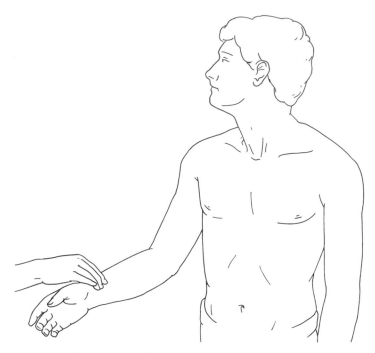

Figure 11–2.   Adson's test. The head is turned toward the examiner and the neck is extended while the arm is at the side, and a deep inspiration is taken. The examiner palpates the radial pulse. The test is positive only if symptoms reported are reproduced. Vascular symptoms are quite rare (see text).

underneath the coracoid process'' (p. 14). In this test, the shoulder is fully abducted and held for 60 seconds while palpating the radial pulse. Reproduction of the symptoms with obliteration of the pulse while simply pushing downward and backward on the clavicle manually, or by the patient bracing his or her shoulders backward (Fig. 11–5), suggests the problem is proximal to the coracoid process, in the costoclavicular space. Other useful clinical tests include a positive Tinel's sign over the part of the brachial plexus affected, reproduction of symptoms with digital pressure in the same area, and reproduction with elevation of the arms to fatigue.

Having a multitude of clinical tests for a single condition is like having many different designs for a knee joint replacement. The more there are, the less confidence should be put in any one of them. With thoracic outlet syndrome, both the diagnosis and management are controversial. As a work-related injury it is rare. It occupies first place in this chapter only by virtue of its proximity to the origin of the

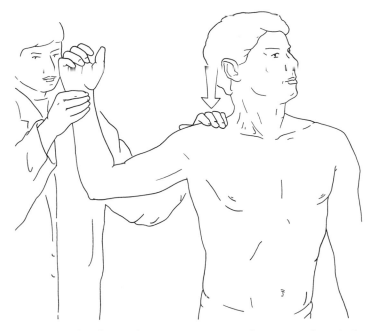

Figure 11–3. Author's quick screening test combines together *A*, the modified Adson's test (the head is *turned away*, neck extended); *B*, 90 degrees of abduction plus external rotation of the shoulder (Roos' test); and *C*, downward pressure on the shoulder while the patient takes a deep breath.

limb. Its complexity makes it impossible to say anything without saying a great deal. The whole subject remains extremely controversial (Lederman, 1987). *Electroneurographic studies* (e.g., somatosensory evoked potentials) may be useful in establishing the diagnosis (Glover et al., 1981). If electrical tests are done, it is essential that the electroneurographer use the "single-purpose" techniques appropriate to the condition, comparing with values obtained in age-matched controls. Technical details are beyond the scope of this book. For a description of such studies, see Sanders and Haug 1991, pp. 88–91).

Musculocutaneous Nerve Entrapment

At the shoulder, the musculocutaneous nerve is at risk where it passes through the coracobrachialis muscle near its origin. A presumptive diagnosis of entrapment was made here in three cases in a study of 146 workers (Ranney et al., 1995). The diagnosis was based on finding tenderness inferior to the coracoid process in these women who had pain, numbness, and/or tingling in the terminal branch of

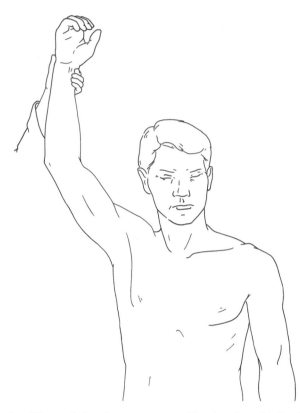

Figure 11–4. Hyperabduction test; specific for brachial plexus stretch around the coracoid process.

the musculocutaneous nerve, namely, the lateral cutaneous nerve of the forearm. Tingling may sometimes be produced in this area by forcefully adducting the arms (e.g., with the hands on the hips), and this helps confirm the diagnosis.

ELBOW AND FOREARM

Cubital Tunnel Syndrome

At the elbow, the *ulnar nerve* passes between the humeral and ulnar heads of the flexor carpi ulnaris, which may be joined by a fibrous band. This is the entrance to the "cubital tunnel." Injury to the ulnar

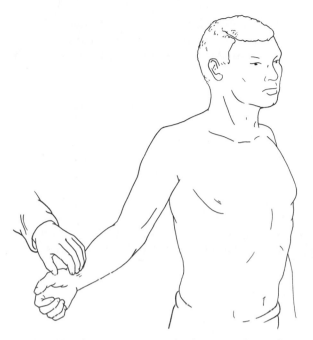

Figure 11–5. Shoulder brace test; specific for costoclavicular compression.

nerve here is called cubital tunnel syndrome. Elbow flexion stretches the ulnar nerve and also narrows the cubital tunnel. Many believe that traction on an ulnar nerve that is impeded from sliding by a fibrous band or bony protruberance is the primary cause of cubital tunnel syndrome. Stretching by more than 8 per cent impedes blood flow in any nerve, a fact well known to clinicians who suture or graft nerves after injury. Although repetitive wrist flexion and ulnar deviation may sometimes be implicated, in fact the problem seems most prevalent in workers who flex their elbows a great deal or lean on them.

Workers with cubital tunnel syndrome will complain of numbness and tingling in the little finger and ulnar border of the forearm. The ulnar nerve will be swollen and tender. If there should be sensory loss distally, it will involve the dorsal as well as volar aspects of the little finger and fifth metacarpal. In severe cases, ulnar-innervated muscles will be weak. Tinel's sign may or may not be present over the ulnar nerve at the elbow. The elbow flexion test is a useful test for examining workers suspected of having this condition. A positive test may reproduce symptoms if the elbow is fully flexed for 60 seconds, with the forearm pronated and the wrist neutral. *As with all provocative tests, it is best not to suggest what symptoms may be provoked but rather say: "Tell me if you feel anything strange."* The elbow flexion test can be made more sensitive if simultaneously there is pressure applied by the examiner's fingers on the ulnar nerve just proximal to the elbow. With this modification, the test was reported to be positive in 91 per cent of 44 elbows with electrodiagnostically proven cubital tunnel syndrome, while only 4 per cent of controls had a false-positive result (Novak et al., 1994).

Subluxation of the Ulnar Nerve

The ulnar nerve may also be traumatized by recurrent subluxation with repetitive elbow motion. In this case, the nerve will be tender and subluxable, but nerve swelling may be minimal. It should be noted that directly touching a normal nerve will cause discomfort, and a comparison with the (it is hoped normal) opposite upper limb should always be made.

Pronator Syndrome

Compression of the median nerve in the elbow region has been given the name pronator syndrome. This is subdivided into pronator teres syndrome (primarily pain and sensory disturbance in the median nerve area) and anterior interosseous nerve syndrome (weakness of forearm muscles supplied by this motor nerve, without sensory loss or tingling). In *pronator teres syndrome*, the site of compression may be proximal or distal to the elbow (see Table 11–3). Just proximal to the elbow, there may be an abnormal development, a supracondylar process arising from the medial supracondylar ridge of the ulna to which is attached the ligament of Struthers. This is quite rare and easily excluded by a plain radiograph. Just distal to the elbow, the bicipital aponeurosis in manual workers (old name: lacertus fibrosis) may be the site of compression. The classic provocative test for compression here is resisted flexion of the elbow with the forearm supinated. In a positive test, there is tingling in the median nerve distribution.

However, by far the majority of work-related compressions of the median nerve in the forearm develop where the median nerve passes through a hypertrophied or swollen pronator teres muscle, or deep to an overused flexor digitorum superficialis (FDS) muscle. If resisted activity of either of these muscles produces tingling in the thumb, the effect is more useful than an immediate nerve conduction study. Of the two, the FDS is more likely to be the source of compression. The technique for stressing the FDS is shown in Chapter 10 (Fig. 10–11).

TABLE 11-3. Median Nerve Compression Syndromes

SYNDROME	SITE OF LESION	TEST	CHARACTERISTIC CLINICAL FEATURES
Carpal tunnel syndrome	Wrist: flexor retinaculum	Phalen's, Lumbrical provocation, Carpal compression	Radial digit numbness,* tingling, pain nocturnally and/ or with wrist flexion/ulnar deviation
Pronator teres syndrome	a. Supracondylar b. Bicipital aponeurosis c. Pronator teres d. Flexor digitorum superficialis (FDS)	a. Radiography b. Flex elbow + supinate forearm c. Resist pronation d. Resist FDS activity (see Fig. 10–11)	Radial digit numbness,* tingling, pain with elbow/ forearm/finger flexion activity that is forceful and repetitive
Anterior interosseous syndrome	Deep branch in forearm	Attempt to form letter "O" with thumb and index finger	Weakness of flexion of thumb and index finger, pain but no numbness

*Pain may extend proximally, but the pattern of numbness reported and any sensory loss there may be on testing must always be confined to an anatomically distinct area distal to the compression site. If numbness extends proximally, consider (1) a more proximal compression in isolation. (2) a more proximal lesion in combination (double-crush phenomenon), or (3) symptom magnification.

Ranney et al. (1995) found the FDS to be compressing the median nerve in 3 of 146 female manual workers doing highly repetitive tasks; no other causes of pronator teres syndrome were seen in this group.

Anterior interosseous nerve syndrome is an entrapment of only this deep motor branch of the median nerve, with resultant weakness or paralysis of the muscles it supplies, namely, the flexor pollicis longus, the flexor digitorum profundus to the index and middle fingers, and the pronator quadratus. There is associated pain but no sensory disturbance. In complete anterior interosseous nerve syndrome, the patient cannot form an "O" with the thumb and index finger. In incomplete lesions, only the thumb long flexor may be affected, and attempting to form an "O" may produce a "D" (see Fig. 11–6).

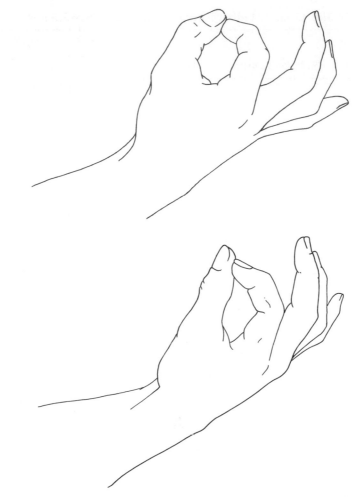

A

B

Figure 11–6. Anterior interosseous nerve paralysis. *A,* Normally an ''O'' can be formed when thumb and fingertips are brought together. *B,* In partial paralysis, the thumb cannot flex at the interphalangeal joint. A ''D'' results. *Illustration continued on opposite page*

Radial Nerve Entrapment

Compression of the radial nerve, like that of the median, may occur at any one of several sites and is similarly divided into two groups, only one of which features paralysis. The purely motor deep branch of the radial nerve may be compressed against the capitellum of the humerus by the overlying extensor carpi radialis brevis (ECRB), before it begins its passage through the supinator muscle. At the entrance to this supinator tunnel, the problem may be a fibrous band,

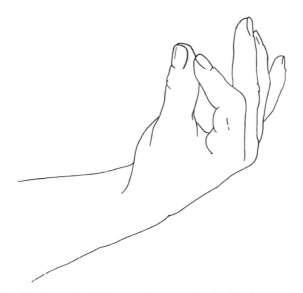

C

Figure 11–6. *Continued* C, In complete paralysis, the flexor digitorum profundus to the index finger is also affected, and therefore flexion of the index distal interphalangeal joint is impossible. This joint may hyperextend slightly because the superficial flexor is not paralyzed. A teardrop-shaped appearance results when attempting an "O."

the arcade of Frohse. Spinner (1968) noted this fibrous band to be present in 30 per cent of the population. Within the tunnel, the deep branch of the radial nerve may be compressed by a supinator muscle that is hypertrophied through overuse.

When there is no muscle paralysis, compression of the radial nerve is called *radial tunnel syndrome*. This is often underdiagnosed or misdiagnosed, and should be considered in anyone with persistent dorsal forearm pain. Workers doing repetitive manual tasks are particularly at risk (Lawrence et al., 1995). The patient usually presents with pain in the extensor region of the forearm brought on or aggravated by forearm rotation. Tenderness over the supinator and pain on resisted supination will confirm the diagnosis. Other suggested provocative tests are of dubious value. These are pain on resisted wrist extension and pain on resisted middle finger extension. One would expect resisted wrist extension to cause pain if that pain is due to compression of the radial nerve deep to the ECRB, either proximal to the supinator tunnel or even within it. However, this test does not distinguish between radial nerve compression and overuse of the ECRB muscle. Pain on resisted middle finger extension that is greater than pain on resisted ring or little finger extension has been listed as a sign of radial tunnel syndrome (Lister, 1977; Mackinnon and Dellon, 1988). Again, one may ask whether this sign excludes local muscle pathology in the digital extensor. Furthermore, the mechanism given for this test is both anatomically and biomechanically unsound.[1]

The entire concept of radial tunnel syndrome merits reappraisal. Results of electromyography and nerve conduction studies are usually normal, and often there is no sign of compression when the nerve is decompressed surgically (Verhaar et al., 1991). In view of recent developments in our understanding of muscle pathology (see Chapter 3), it is possible that pain relief after surgery may be due to muscle decompression, and the radial nerve never was at risk.

If there is dorsal forearm pain only and no paralysis, but the pain can be relieved by anesthetic infiltration of the radial nerve, there is general agreement among hand surgeons that the diagnosis of radial tunnel syndrome has been confirmed. This entrapment of the radial nerve is believed to be one of the main causes of "tennis elbow" that fails to respond to conservative treatment. An operation to explore the radial nerve is then undertaken, and this usually is accompanied by release of the common extensor origin. However, it remains to be determined whether many of those patients diagnosed as having radial tunnel syndrome might in fact have simply a chronic muscle fatigue problem, which also could be helped by this operative procedure, the postoperative rest that follows, or both.

Radial nerve entrapment in the forearm with paralysis is a different problem altogether. This is called *posterior interosseous nerve syndrome* (see Table 11–4). When the deep branch of the radial nerve exits from the supinator muscle, its name changes and it becomes the posterior interosseous nerve. This nerve supplies (among others) the deep outcropping muscles of the thumb and the extensor indicis proprius. Weakness of the index extensor will confirm the diagnosis: The index finger cannot be held straight when resistance is applied with the other fingers fully flexed (T. Wadsworth, 1987, personal communication).

---

[1]Mosley et al. (1991) offered the usual explanation that ECRB activity is increased in resisted middle finger extension more so than with adjacent fingers because it inserts into the third metacarpal (to which the middle finger attaches). But the middle finger extensor does not arise from the third metacarpal. Furthermore, when finger extension is resisted without supporting the wrist as shown by Mosley et al. (1991) in their Figure 39, this creates a flexor movement at the wrist that would require ECRB activity to resist it. However, a similar flexor moment is created in resisting *any* finger. When the ECRB is called into activity, the magnitude of the force it creates is proportional to the amount of resistance and to the distance from the center of rotation at the wrist. This distance will be shorter on a shorter finger. Thus the pain felt in an injured ECRB will be greater when resisting extension of a long finger than a shorter finger. This test tells us nothing about radial tunnel syndrome unless chronic injury to the ECRB can be excluded.

TABLE 11–4. Radial Nerve Compression Syndromes

Syndrome	Site of Lesion	Test	Characteristic Clinical Features
Wartenberg's syndrome	Superficial radial nerve	Flex and ulnar deviate wrist, forearm pronated	Pain, numbness, tingling in dorsum of thumb, index fingers, hand
Radial tunnel syndrome	a. ECRB/capit. b. Fibrous band c. In supinator	a. Resisted wrist extension* c. Resisted supination	Pain in radial nerve area with no sensory loss, related to repetitive forearm and wrist movement
Posterior interosseous syndrome	Deep branch anywhere in supinator	Resisted index finger extension	Pain without sensory loss, as above, but with weakness of thumb and index finger extensors

ECRB/capit. = between extensor carpi radialis brevis and capitellum.
*Pain on resisted wrist extension is considered by many a good test, but not so by this author.

WRIST AND HAND

Carpal Tunnel Syndrome

Carpal tunnel syndrome, or compression of the median nerve at the wrist, may result from hypertrophic synovium as a consequence of repetitive finger motion (Schuind et al., 1990). The compression site is most frequently the *distal edge* of the transverse carpal ligament (Nathan et al., 1990), also known as the flexor retinaculum. This suggests that hypertrophied lumbrical muscles could be impinging on the median nerve, acting as the ultimate or "last straw." During carpal tunnel release, Yii and Elliott (1994) noted in 32 patients that, although fewer than 20 per cent had any part of a lumbrical muscle in the tunnel on finger extension, all lumbricals except those of two little fingers had moved into the tunnel on full finger flexion. Similar findings are reported by Cobb et al. (1994). Because the primary role of the lumbrical is to draw the profundus tendon distally on finger extension (Ranney and Wells, 1988), workers who repetitively flex their fingers will develop hypertrophied lumbricals in concert with hypertrophy of the profundus muscle. These larger than normal lumbricals, on finger flexion, could possibly constitute yet another compressive force in the development of carpal tunnel syndrome (Ranney, 1996b).

Both clinical and epidemiologic studies have also implicated wrist movements and deviant wrist postures as etiologic factors. Even Phalen's provocative test for this condition requires acute wrist flexion. Having cited repetitive motion and posture as causative factors, it must be noted that overuse at work is only one factor contributing to the development of carpal tunnel syndrome. Others include overuse at home (e.g., knitting), rheumatoid and osteoarthritis, trauma (e.g., Colles' fracture), gout, diabetes mellitus, renal failure, vitamin B_6 deficiency, Paget's disease, pregnancy, and other changes in the hormonal environment (e.g., menstrual cycle variations, hypothyroidism, and disorders of the pituitary gland). Even age alone has been implicated. However, if we look at various industries whose workers are exposed to repetitive finger and wrist movement, we see a direct correlation between these risk factors and the prevalence of carpal tunnel syndrome. Silverstein et al. (1987) found that, when high force and high repetition were combined, the odds ratio for getting carpal tunnel syndrome was more than 15 compared to low-force/low-repetitive jobs. They found that, of these two factors, high repetition (e.g., a cycle time of <30 seconds) was the more important. This is in keeping with the later findings by Schuind et al. (1990) of synovial thickening of finger flexor tendons, a pathologic change one would expect to occur as a result of repetition-induced friction.

Tests for carpal tunnel syndrome include sensory and motor assessment, Phalen's test, Tinel's sign, the carpal compression test, the lumbrical provocation test, and nerve conduction studies. Phalen's test is performed by fully flexing the wrist passively and noting if tingling occurs in the thumb, lateral fingers, or both within 1 or 2 minutes (Busquets, 1993). This test may be reinforced and thus made more sensitive by asking the patient to actively press the thumb and index finger together at the same time. Tinel's sign (or the Hoffman-Tinel sign) is positive when, on tapping with the end of a finger over any nerve, there is a tingle in the distribution of that nerve. It was devised to determine the end-point of regenerating axoplasm after nerve suture. It is therefore not surprising to find that it is often negative at the point of constriction of a nerve. If positive, Tinel's sign aids the diagnosis; if negative, it means nothing. Direct digital pressure over the distal edge of the flexor retinaculum for 30 seconds will frequently reproduce symptoms (Durkan, 1991). This "carpal compression test" was found to be more sensitive and more specific than either Phalen's test or Tinsel's sign. Clenching the fist for 60 seconds (the lumbrical provocation test) reproduces the patient's symptoms (Yii and Elliott, 1994) when positive.

Nerve electrodiagnostic tests that confirm the clinical diagnosis are always helpful. If negative, they should stimulate a renewed search for pathology elsewhere (Payan, 1988). However, nerve conduction tests can be normal in the presence of mild carpal tunnel syndrome. Grundberg (1983) operated on 32 wrists based on a clinical diagnosis of carpal tunnel syndrome when the nerve conduction tests were negative, and 31 were relieved by division of the flexor retinaculum. Grundberg's experience has cast doubt on the concept that nerve conduction studies are "the gold standard" for diagnosis. The diagnosis must primarily be made on a wise synthesis of history and physical findings. In those patients with a clear clinical diagnosis but negative nerve tests, temporary relief of symptoms with cortisone injection provides adequate confirmation.

In defense of the gold standard, it must be acknowledged that today there are more sophisticated electroneurographic tests for diagnosing carpal tunnel syndrome. Routine tests will reveal much valuable information of a general nature. However, if these are negative, single-purpose studies (in this case specific to carpal tunnel syndrome) must be employed (e.g., comparing median and ulnar nerve characteristics). In this way, the number of false negatives will be drastically reduced. Today's injured workers are also more sophisticated, and may be able to give a convincing history after reading it in a book or being coached by an advisor. The possibility of a false-negative objective test must be carefully weighed against a suspected false-positive clinical picture.

A special warning is required before leaving the topic of carpal tunnel syndrome. Ranney et al.'s (1995) study of 146 workers indicated many workers have multiple coexisting problems. Operations for carpal tunnel syndrome are much less successful in workers than in those patients in whom it is considered not to be work related. It could be that in some of these workers there were other problems. So when making the popular diagnosis of carpal tunnel syndrome, the examiner must determine whether there are other injuries also.

Ulnar Carpal Tunnel Syndrome

The term "ulnar carpal tunnel syndrome" refers to entrapment of the ulnar nerve at the wrist in what is known as Guyon's canal.[2]

---

[2]This canal is a small tube enclosing the ulnar nerve and artery. These structures cross the wrist superficial to the transverse carpal ligament, not deep to it as the median nerve does. The volar carpal ligament forms the roof of Guyon's canal. The floor is the transverse carpal ligament, known also as the flexor retinaculum (Hollinshead, 1982).

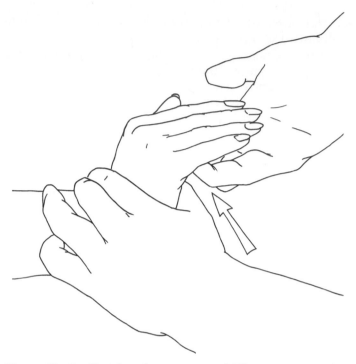

Figure 11–7. Test for ulnar nerve and T1 root compression.

Continued low-level pressure here will bring it on. This is a well-recognized problem in cyclists; it may also occur as a result of intermittent impact (see Hypothenar Hammer Syndrome later in this section). Repetitive wrist flexion and extension and the use of vibrating tools have also been implicated. The effect of ulnar nerve compression at the wrist is most often purely motor, with possible paralysis of all intrinsic muscles of the fingers except the first two lumbricals.[3] Alternatively, there may be just sensory loss, or a combination of the two. This author's test for ulnar nerve (and also first thoracic nerve root) function is shown in Figure 11–7. Other tests include palpating for tenderness over Guyon's canal and a positive Tinel's sign at this point. Ulnar carpal tunnel syndrome may be mistaken clinically for (median) carpal tunnel syndrome. Given the current popularity of carpal tunnel syndrome as a cause of work-related distress, it is more likely that median nerve entrapment will be suspected, when really

---

[3]This pattern of paralysis contrasts sharply with that of thoracic outlet syndrome, in which (when severe enough to cause paralysis) the thenar muscles are usually primarily affected. This can happen because all small muscles of the hand are innervated by the first thoracic nerve root. However, the ulnar nerve does not supply the thenar muscles, nor the index and middle finger lumbrical muscles.

it may be the ulnar nerve that somewhere along its course is in difficulty (see Table 11–5).

Wartenberg's Syndrome

Wartenberg's syndrome is entrapment of the purely sensory superficial radial nerve deep to the brachioradialis. When present, pain, tingling, and possibly numbness are reported over the dorsum of the thumb, the index finger, and related areas of the hand and distal forearm. Tinel's sign may be positive over the course of this nerve, which lies subcutaneously over bone proximal to the radial styloid process. A useful provocative test consists of holding the wrist flexed and ulnar deviated with the forearm in full pronation for 1 minute (Dellon and Mackinnon, 1986). Pain and tingling occur as the nerve is compressed between the brachioradialis and the adjacent ECRB. These symptoms may also occur with resisted wrist extension. Finkelstein's test and even simple wrist flexion may be painful, and therefore Wartenberg's syndrome should be considered when such are found.

Vibration White Finger

Vibration white finger is the chief vascular problem seen as a result of industrial overuse. Vibrating tools also distort the perception of position sense so that grip force is almost doubled (Radwin et al., 1987). This is one cause of muscle fatigue and associated pain. The neurophysiologic reason is that vibration-induced spindle stimulation leads higher centers to act as though the muscle fibers are longer than they really are (Goodwin et al., 1972). If occurring over a long period of time, vibration can also cause permanent vascular insufficiency.

TABLE 11–5. Differential Diagnosis of Fifth Digit Numbness/Tingling

Ulnar carpal tunnel syndrome
Vibration white finger
Cubital tunnel syndrome
Thoracic outlet syndrome
C8 pressure for other reasons
Anxiety plus work-related pain
Peripheral neuritis
Hypothenar hammer syndrome
Vasculitis (e.g., diabetes)
Carpal tunnel syndrome in a poor historian

The end result is poor circulation, and because the nerves also are deprived of good blood supply, sensory innervation is also disturbed.

Vibration white finger is characterized by numbness and temporary blanching of the affected finger(s) when exposed to the cold in workers exposed to prolonged vibration in the range of 40 to 200 Hz. It is a form of secondary Raynaud's phenomenon. However, Boyle et al. (1988) report 12 of 19 patients with vibration white finger as having episodes of numbness and tingling *not* associated with pallor, whose "history and physical signs were consistent with carpal tunnel syndrome" (p. 172). In fact, both conditions may be seen together in the same individual (Savage et al., 1990). Thus, even though it is much less common than carpal tunnel syndrome, vibration white finger must be included in the differential diagnosis when assessing any worker with a sensory disturbance in the hand, and be a primary consideration if the worker uses vibrating tools.

Hypothenar Hammer Syndrome

Hypothenar hammer syndrome is the picturesque name given to the condition that results when the base of the hypothenar region is used like the head of a hammer. The ulnar artery within Guyon's canal is damaged by repetitive trauma. A thrombus results, blocking the artery. The resultant swelling may be enough to also compress the ulnar nerve. Symptoms may include pain, tingling, numbness in the litter finger, cold intolerance, and pallor.

On examination of the base of the hypothenar area, a mass is often palpable. A positive Allen's test is diagnostic. This test is performed as follows. Both the radial and ulnar pulses are located, then compressed simultaneously. The hand is opened and shut a few times to remove venous and capillary blood, leaving the hand quite pale. Releasing the radial artery first allows the palm to quickly become pink. Then the procedure is repeated and the ulnar artery is released while the radial remains compressed. In normal hands, the return of color will be slower on releasing the ulnar artery than on releasing the radial because it is a smaller artery. However, the hand should become pink in a few seconds, and as quickly as it does on the opposite side. In a positive test, the affected palm remains pale for a longer duration than normal.

Focal Dystonia

Focal dystonia, seen in musicians and workers, has been described as a painless loss of coordination in which the desired movements are replaced by undesired ones (Fry, 1991). These movements may be counterproductive, such as the little and ring fingers curling under when all fingers are extended to reach out and grasp a musical instrument, or inability to strike a typewriter key. Tremor and disordered sequence of movement may occur. Although dystonia is relatively more prevalent in musicians, it also may be seen in nonmusicians performing repetitive manual tasks, such as writers (Sheehy and Marsden, 1982).

The pathology seems to lie within the central nervous system. Electromyographic studies by Cohen and Hallet (1982) have shown longer than normal bursts of activity in agonists and co-contraction in antagonists. Newmark and Hochberg (1987) have demonstrated inhibition of H reflexes, giving further evidence of structural changes within the spinal cord. Fry (1988) suggested "the abnormality may lie in the supraspinal influences on the spinal cord rather than in the cord itself" (p. 909). What was once considered to be just a peripheral phenomenon initiates changes centrally that then perpetuate the peripheral manifestation. This is a process similar to that which takes place in patients with chronic pain.

REFERENCES

Adson AW, Coffey JR: Cervical rib: A method of anterior approach for relief of symptoms by division of the scalenus anticus. Ann Surg 85:839–857, 1927.

Anson BJ: Morris' Human Anatomy, 12th ed. New York, McGraw-Hill, 1966, p 46.

Boyle JC, Smith NJ, Burke FD: Vibration white finger. J Hand Surg 13B:171–176, 1988.

Busquets MAV: Historical commentary: The wrist flexion test (Phalen's sign). J Hand Surg 19A:521, 1993.

Cobb TK, An K-N, Cooney WP, et al: Lumbrical muscle incursion into the carpal tunnel during finger flexion. J Hand Surg 19B:434–438, 1994.

Cohen LG, Hallet M: Hand cramps: Clinical features and electromyographic patterns in a focal dystonia. Neurology 38:1005, 1988.

Cuetter AC, Bartoszek MD: The thoracic outlet syndrome: Controversies, overdiagnosis, overtreatment and recommendations for management. Muscle Nerve 12:410–419, 1989.

Dellon AL, Mackinnon SE: Radial sensory nerve entrapment in the forearm. J Hand Surg 11A:199–205, 1986.

Durkan JA: A new diagnostic test for carpal tunnel syndrome. J Bone Joint Surg 73A:535–538, 1991.

Fry JH: Focal dystonia (occupational cramp) masquerading as nerve entrapment or hysteria. Plast Reconstr Surg 82:908–910, 1988.

Fry JH: The effect of overuse on musician's technique: A comparative and historical review. Int J Arts Med 1:46–55, 1991.

Glover JL, Werth RM, Bendick PJ, et al: Evoked responses in the diagnosis of thoracic outlet syndrome. Surgery 89:86–93, 1981.

Goodwin GM, McCloskey DI, Mattews BC: Proprioceptive illusions induced by muscle vibration: Contribution by muscle spindles to perception? Science 175:1382–1384, 1972.

Grundberg AB: Carpal tunnel decompression in spite of normal electromyography. J Hand Surg 8:348–349, 1983.

Hollinshead WH: Anatomy for Surgeons, Vol. 3. Philadelphia, Harper & Row, 1982, pp 389, 472.

Karas SE: Thoracic outlet syndrome. Clin Sport Med 9:297–310, 1990.

Lawrence T, Mobbs P, Fortems Y, et al: Radial tunnel syndrome. J Hand Surg 20B:454–459, 1995.

Lederman RJ: Thoracic outlet syndrome: Review of the controversies and a report of 17 instrumental musicians. Med Probl Perform Art 2:87–91, 1987.

Leffert RD: Thoracic outlet syndrome and the shoulder. Clin Sports Med 2: 439–452, 1983.

Lister GD: The Hand: Diagnosis and Indications. Edinburgh, Churchill-Livingstone, 1977.

Mackinnon SE, Dellon AL: Multiple crush syndrome. In Mackinnon SE, Dellon AL (eds): Surgery of the Peripheral Nerve. New York, Thieme Medical, 1988, pp 360–368.

Mosley LH, Kalafut RM, Levinson PD, et al: Cumulative trauma disorders and compression neuropathies of the upper extremities. In Kasdan ML (ed): Occupational Hand and Upper Extremity Injuries & Diseases. Philadelphia, Hanley & Belfus, 1991, pp 353–402.

Nathan PA, Srinivasan H, Doyle LS, et al: Location of impaired sensory conduction of the median nerve in carpal tunnel syndrome. J Hand Surg 15B: 89–92, 1990.

Newmark J, Hochberg FH: Isolated painless manual incoordination in 57 musicians. J Neurol Neurosurg Psychiatry 50:291–295, 1987.

Novak CB, Lee GW, Mackinnon SE, et al: Provocative testing for cubital tunnel syndrome. J Hand Surg 19A:817–820, 1994.

Payan J: The carpal tunnel syndrome: Can we do better? J Hand Surg 13B: 365–367, 1988.

Peet RM, Henriksen JD, Anderson TP, et al: Thoracic outlet syndrome: Evaluation of a therapeutic exercise program. Staff Meet Mayo Clinic 31:281–287, 1956.

Radwin RC, Armstrong TJ, Chaffin DB: Power hand tool vibration effects on grip exertions. Ergonomics 30:833–839, 1987.

Ranney DA: The thoracic outlet: An anatomical re-definition that makes clinical sense. Clin Anat 9:50–52, 1996a.

Ranney DA: Letter to the editor. J Hand Surg 21A:152, 1996b.

Ranney DA, Wells RP: Lumbrical muscle function as revealed by a new and physiological approach. Anat Rec 222:110–114, 1988.

Ranney DA, Wells RP, Moore A: Upper limb musculoskeletal disorders in highly repetitive industries: Precise anatomical physical findings. Ergonomics 38:1408–1423, 1995.

Roos DB, Owens JC: Thoracic outlet syndrome. Arch Surg 93:71–74, 1966.

Sanders RJ, Haug CE: Thoracic Outlet Syndrome: A Common Sequela of Neck Injuries. Philadelphia, JB Lippincott, 1991.

Savage R, Burke FD, Smith NJ, et al: Carpal tunnel syndrome in association with vibration white finger. J Hand Surg 15B:100–103, 1990.

Schuind F, Ventura M, Pasteels JL: Idiopathic carpal tunnel syndrome: Histologic study of flexor tendon synovium. J Hand Surg 15A:497–503, 1990.

Sheehy MP, Marsden CD: Writer's cramp—a focal dystonia. Brain 105:461–480, 1982.

Silverstein BA, Fine LJ, Armstrong TJ: Occupational factors and carpal tunnel syndrome. Am J Ind Med *11*:343–358, 1987.

Spinner M: The arcade of Frohse and its relationship to posterior interosseous nerve paralysis. J Bone Joint Surg *50B*:809–812, 1968.

Travell JG, Simons DG: Myofascial Pain and Dysfunction: The Trigger Point Manual, Vol 1. Baltimore, Williams & Wilkins, 1983, p 355.

Verhaar J, Spaans F: Radial tunnel syndrome: An investigation of compression neuropathy as a possible cause. J Bone Joint surg *73A*:539–544, 1991.

Wilbourn AJ: Thoracic outlet syndrome surgery causing severe brachial plexopathy. Muscle Nerve *11*:66–74, 1988.

Wright IS: The neurovascular syndrome produced by hyperabduction of the arms. Am Heart J *29*:1–19, 1945.

Yii NW, Elliot D: A study of the dynamic relationship of the lumbrical muscles in the carpal tunnel. J Hand Surg *19B*:439–443, 1994.

12
Establishing a Prognosis for Low Back Problems

Michel Rossignol

IMPORTANCE OF PROGNOSIS

The establishment of a prognosis in workers with low back pain is a key element in the prevention of chronicity and recurrences, which account for three quarters of the disability and compensation costs. This chapter is based on the epidemiologic literature and presents scientific data that have been demonstrated to have prognostic value regarding the risk of chronicity of low back pain. This information is presented in complement to Chapter 9 on clinical diagnosis, in order to broaden the scope of evaluation of workers who have been disabled for 2 to 3 months following a back injury. When considering duration of disability, *past injuries are included* in the cumulative total.

In medicine, it takes 10 to 15 years to establish a change in treatment methods. Such changes seem to depend more on how new drugs and management approaches are marketed than on the quality of the scientific evidence that would support such changes. The multiplication of diagnostic and therapeutic modalities and devices have oriented back pain sufferers toward the traditional approach of "seeking a cure." However, numerous studies in the past 15 years have demonstrated that, for the majority of back pain sufferers, the active participation of the patient in the therapy is the key element to recovery and to prevention of recurrences. This idea is certainly not new. In the 1950s, Karl Hirsch, a Swedish orthopedic surgeon, had recognized the limitations of surgery in helping people with back pain and was advocating what he called "conservative approaches." By this he meant not only nonsurgical methods, but also a close interactive process between the physician, the patient, and the back pain problem (Hirsch, 1971).

When epidemiologic studies of back pain were begun in the early 1980s, the prevalent attitude was that back pain was not a serious medical problem for the vast majority of patients. Indeed, once a specialized consultant had ruled out a serious condition and had advocated continuing "conservative treatment," the precise diagnosis of what had caused the back pain was not considered important at all. This concept seems a contradiction to what had always been taught in medicine: that the basis of any treatment was a precise diagnosis. In fact, in back pain, the making of the diagnosis is more than a basis for treatment; it can be the beginning of the treatment itself (Waddell, 1987).

The current recommendations for management of back pain first focus on the identification of "red flags" (conditions requiring urgent treatment) (Agency for Health Care Policy and Research, 1994; Spitzer et al., 1987). After these conditions have been ruled out, a conservative approach is advocated for those 90 per cent of back pain patients whose pain is "nonspecific." Until the late 1980s, we had only a vague notion of what conservative therapy meant, but the concept of a back school had already existed for 30 years (White, 1992). Several clinicians and researchers have recognized the importance of defining the conservative approach (Mayer et al., 1987; Nachemson, 1992), whereas others have demonstrated the lack of efficacy, in randomized controlled trials, of commonly used therapies that can therefore no longer be considered conservative, such as bed rest and transcutaneous electrical nerve stimulation (Deyo et al., 1986, 1990; Malmivaara et al., 1995). Paradoxically, although the concept of active physical treatment for back pain is becoming better defined, little scientific work has been done on the diagnosis of back pain.

The prognosis of back pain lies within a delicate balance of two goals, establishing a new paradigm:

1. To seek out conditions (red flags) that require specific and urgent treatment (surgical or otherwise).

2. To avoid the seemingly endless pursuit of searching for a cause, a search that would not benefit the patient and could interfere with an active participation in therapy.

The balance is fragile because, once the focus has been put on the first goal, it becomes difficult to switch to the second, from the patient's perspective, and it might be difficult to orient the treatment toward recovery rather than toward finding a cure. The next five sections are presented to help establish a prognosis for back pain, and concern equally what has been called until now specific and nonspecific low back pain. First, however, some key words must be defined.

Definition of Key Terms

Prognosis (also called the outcome in epidemiologic research) is usually measured in terms of (1) time to functional recovery (i.e., return to work or to usual activities), and (2) periods of recurrence with a functional deficit, within a certain period of time of follow-up (anything between a few weeks to a few years).

Return to work, in this chapter, corresponds to the date when a worker returns to the same occupation he or she had before the back-related disability, or to another regular job. This point of reference for the calculation of the time to functional recovery tries to avoid the bias caused by administrative pressure to return to a temporary assignment (light duty), which differs among workplaces and insurance carriers (Butler et al., 1995).

Recurrence, in a general sense, is any period of disability caused by back pain that follows a period of return to work after a back-related problem. This is so whether or not those periods are considered a recurrence by administrative definitions. Recurrences are more frequent in the first year following an episode (Rossignol et al., 1992), but there is theoretically no time limit in the definition of recurrence because a history of back problem, at any time in the past, is a risk factor for future episodes.

Back disability is the incapacity to accomplish, because of a back problem, a task that is normally carried out. The back problem might be pain, physical impairment (e.g., an inability to bend forward), or both. When the capacity to accomplish a task falls short of societal expectations (e.g., as a worker, spouse, sports participant), it is termed a handicap (Waddell, 1992).

Epidemiologic proof, as applied in this chapter, is an evaluation of the degree of usefulness of diagnostic aids through population studies. The strength of proof depends on the type of study, the choice of the study population, and the level of control of potential sources of bias. The Quebec Task Force on activity-related spinal disorders classified epidemiologic proof in five categories (Spitzer et al., 1987). They are, in *descending order of strength*

1. Usefulness demonstrated by randomized controlled trial
2. Usefulness demonstrated by nonrandomized controlled trial
3. Contraindicated on the basis of scientific evidence

4. Common practice but no supporting scientific evidence
5. Not in common practice and no scientific evidence

Validity of instruments used for assessing the functional limitations of patients with low back pain has been addressed primarily with the following measurements:

1. *Reliability:* the extent to which the instrument gives the same result when administered under similar conditions
2. *Internal consistency:* the extent to which related questions give similar answers
3. *Responsiveness*, also called sensitivity to change: the extent to which the result will differ when the instrument is administered to patients in different clinical stages of severity
4. *Criterion validity:* the extent to which the measurement given by the instrument correlates with other measures of back-related problems

ASSESSING RED FLAGS

All specialists of the musculoskeletal system agree that there are a few conditions associated with back pain that require urgent intervention. Although rare, their potential presence can be easily recognized by the nonspecialist and they should never be overlooked. Spine fracture, tumor, infection, and cauda equina syndrome have characteristic features regarding history of development, symptoms, and signs that should raise red flags of warning. Table 12–1 summarizes these and is based on recommendations made by the Agency for Health Care Policy and Research (AHCPR) (1994).

A short questionnaire including all these items should be part of the initial interview with a patient with back pain, even if this is not the first visit to a health care practitioner for the condition. The suspicion of one of these conditions requires immediate referral to the appropriate specialist. The identification of red flags requires a complete review of systems and a complete physical examination at the first contact with a patient.

PAIN ASSESSMENT

Mode of Onset and Time Elapsed since Injury

Pain is the chief complaint bringing back pain patients to consult. It is therefore the starting point in the establishment of a diagnosis

TABLE 12–1. Red Flags Indicating Urgent Intervention Required*

CONDITION	HISTORY, SYMPTOMS, AND SIGNS
Fracture	Major trauma such as fall from a height Trauma in older persons, potentially osteoporotic patient
Tumor	Age over 50 or under 20 History of cancer Unexplained weight loss Recent fever or chills Pain worsens when supine; severe night pain

Infection	History of recent infection
	Recent fever or chills
	Reduction in immunity level, such as
	  Current use of oral steroids
	  Organ transplant
	  Intravenous drug abuse
	  Human immunodeficiency virus infection

Cauda equina
  syndrome
	Saddle anesthesia
	Recent onset of urinary incontinence or
	  retention
	Major weakness in knee extension and ankle
	  dorsiflexors (foot drop)
	Anal sphincter laxity on digital rectal
	  examination

*From Bigos S, Bowyer O, Braen G, et al: *Acute Low Back Problems in Adults* (Clinical Practice Guideline, Quick Reference Number 14) Publication Number 95-0643. Agency for Health Care Policy and Research, 1994. This document is in the public domain and may be used and reprinted without special permission.

and of the doctor-patient relationship. Learning details about the pain is the first step in assessment of a back problem (Table 12–2). The *history of onset* of the current problem will reveal whether there was an accidental event associated with an acute onset of the pain, versus a gradual development.

In the *acute-onset back pain* related to an accidental event, the nature of the event, such as a fall from a height, brings to mind the possi-

TABLE 12–2. Assessment of Back
Problems in Workers

I	Pain
II	Physical signs
III	Functional status
IV	Return-to-work status

bility of a fracture, which should be investigated right away. Fortunately, the majority of accidental events reported in the workplace are associated with *less severe injuries* related to strenuous efforts or false movements, which involve enough energy to cause only soft tissue injuries.

It has been estimated that up to one third of soft tissue injuries reported as being associated with an accidental event (acute onset) in the workplace are in fact back problems that had evolved over a period of days or weeks (Hadler, 1987; Manning et al., 1984). We should therefore not be satisfied with only the description of an acute event; we should question the patient about back pain status in the week preceding the event. Although there are clinicians who believe that a gradual onset confers a poorer prognosis than an acute onset, there is no scientific evidence, to this date, to support such a view. The real importance of making this distinction is rather for the clinician to be able to count the total number of days that the patient has experienced pain in the current episode. This information is crucial because the further away the date of onset of the problem is from its assessment, the greater is the risk of developing a chronic state (Rossignol et al., 1992; Spitzer et al., 1987).

The management guidelines use the *time elapsed* from the onset as a reference for orienting health care. The following landmarks have been used:

1. *Acute phase:* first and second weeks
2. *Subacute phase:* third through sixth weeks
3. *Prechronicization period:* seventh and eighth weeks
4. *Chronicization period:* third through sixth months
5. *Chronic phase:* sixth month and beyond

Previous History

In the same way that time elapsed since injury is a predictor of chronicity, a previous experience with back pain, especially in the previous year, is a factor that has been consistently associated with a risk of recurrence and of chronicity. Whether or not the current episode is considered by the patient or by the health care practitioner as a recurrence from a previous episode does not matter in this respect. The cumulative number of days of back pain causing an incapacity (at work or otherwise) in the past year must be included to determine the duration of the current episode with regard to the risk of chronicity. Rossignol et al. (1992) suggested that a cumulative duration of 3 months of disability from work, *including the current and past year episodes*, places a patient in a chronicization phase.

Pain Distribution

Another key factor in establishing the prognosis of back pain is the distribution of the pain. The Quebec Task Force suggested three categories for distribution of pain:

1. Pain localized to the back
2. Pain radiating down the leg but above the knee
3. Pain radiating down the leg, below the knee

There is some epidemiologic evidence that severe sciatic pain (third category) represents a risk of chronicity (Weber et al., 1993). Sciatic pain, long considered a sign of nerve root irritation, is often not accompanied by neurologic signs and is not, in itself, a reason to order specialized imaging tests in the acute and subacute phases. However, it is important as a predictor of chronicity.

Intensity and Character

The change in character and severity of the pain since the onset is an important clue to the anticipated recovery pattern of a patient. An improvement in symptoms, even modest and of short duration, is an indication that the problem has started to resolve. Back pain recovery may follow an irregular pattern, periods of partial recovery being interspersed with exacerbations. This saw-toothed recovery pattern can be superimposed on the classic epidemiologic recovery curve (Spitzer et al., 1987), because the rate of recovery of one particular patient does not necessarily follow a smooth curve (Fig. 12–1). It is useful to instruct the patient about the meaning of the symptoms within the context of recovery, because relapses, which are so typical of back pain, can be mistaken for an aggravation of the condition, which could lead to worries and loss of confidence in the diagnosis and treatment.

The *intensity* of back pain is best assessed by using a visual analog scale on which the patient indicates by a mark on a graduated 10-cm line the intensity of pain relative to the worst pain ever felt (back pain, toothache, headache, etc.). This instrument has shown good intrasubject reliability and can be used to follow pain intensity in a patient from one visit to the next (Melzack and Wall, 1982). Because the intensity of pain can change dramatically in the interval between visits, the patient can be provided with a pain calendar on which every change can be recorded with the date. The establishment of the recovery profile by the patient outside the medical office is a valuable tool to both monitor recovery and delegate to the patient part of the pain management.

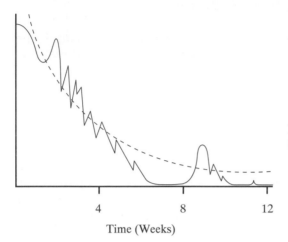

Figure 12–1. Pattern of recovery.

Time (Weeks)

- - - - : Recovery pattern from epidemiologic studies
——— : Recovery pattern of a hypothetical case

The *character* of the pain is best assessed in primary care with a pain drawing (Ransford et al., 1976). The patient will take only minutes to fill this out, and it provides the clinician with a rough screening assessment of the "suffering" component of pain. *Suffering is important to identify early, because it can constitute an important barrier to recovery.*

Health Care Product Utilization

Back pain can be monitored by identifying the amount of health care that a patient has sought: nature and number of diagnostic tests and consultations, number of pills taken, number of visits to back specialists, number and nature of manual and physiotherapeutic treatments, and nonprescription therapies such as back belts and braces, magnets, and homeopathic and naturopathic products, among others. A thorough questionnaire is important to identify early the patients who have a problem with analgesic abuse, or who seem to depend too much on others for pain management.

As the health care practitioner is aware, a wealth of products are offered on the market for back pain sufferers. Most of them have never been tested for efficacy and some have been shown to be of no utility at all. The patient who does not understand the diagnostic process and the natural history of back pain will have a weak relation with the clinician, and eventually will consult elsewhere. Knowledge of the pattern of health services and product utilization is important in establishing prognosis; it gives an idea of the strength of the patient-clinician relationship. The patient should be encouraged, when appropriate, to read up on the topic of back pain. There are several excellent books accessible to the general public. This is another way the patient can take an active role in the health management process.

PHYSICAL SIGNS

Physical examination of the patient with low back pain involves a systematic review of the spine, the sacroiliac and hip joints, and the lower extremities; a neurologic examination, with a search for signs of nerve root compression; and examination of the abdomen, including the digital rectal examination. There are excellent audiovisual programs that review the examination of a patient with low back pain. Those who do not specialize in musculoskeletal problems should review such programs once a year (see also Chapter 9). This section discusses the elements of the physical examination that have been mentioned in epidemiologic studies.

Height and Weight

Increased height has been associated with back pain (Yu et al., 1984), possibly through an increased stress on the discs (Kelsey, 1976). However, contrary to what would be expected, the results of studies on obesity have *not* been consistent. This is not to say that weight is not important, because excessive weight can be a barrier to doing the exercises in the treatment plan. Height is an element that adds to the suspicion of a disc problem in the presence of signs of nerve root compression, but is by no mean a firm prognostic indicator. Overall, height and weight are not primary prognostic factors but can be important determinants of therapeutic outcome, although a literature review found no study that looked at this specifically.

Scoliosis

Another anthropometric observation is the presence of scoliosis. Although the radiologic presence of scoliosis has not been convincingly associated with back pain in some studies (Gibson, 1988), the study of a cohort of adolescent patients with idiopathic scoliosis followed through adult life showed that they had significantly more back pain than matched controls. The type of treatment and the degree of curvature did not seem to modify that association (Mayo et al., 1994). Little is known about the pathogenesis of back pain among adolescents with scoliosis, but it seems that a history of back pain at that age, whether a diagnosis of scoliosis was made or not, might be a predictor of back pain later in life. The reason a history of back pain in adolescence is a predictor of back pain later in life remains unknown, but its prognostic value, described among adults, could also be true among adolescents, independent of the diagnosis of scoliosis.

Schober Test

The single measurement of spinal movement that has shown sufficient reliability and responsiveness to be considered for use in clinical trials is the Schober test (MacRae and Wright, 1969; Schober, 1937). This is explained in part by the facts that it is easy to measure and is more specific to the lumbar motion than other indicators, such as the finger-floor distance or goniometer measurements. It should be mentioned, however, that a decrease of motion, measured in degrees, is claimed by many practitioners to be associated with a specific type of spinal lesion and a specific prognosis, but there is no epidemiologic proof of such at present. The Schober test or the modified Schober test (MacRae and Wright, 1969) should always be performed when examining a patient with low back pain (Fig. 12–2).

Signs of Nerve Root Compression

All the current clinical guidelines use the presence of signs of nerve root compression to orient the diagnostic and therapeutic interventions. Like sciatic pain, other signs of nerve root compression are considered to indicate that specialized imaging, electrodiagnostic tests, or consultations with a specialist of the musculoskeletal system are needed. However, such interventions, in the absence of red flags, are not advisable before 4 to 7 weeks after the onset of pain, and then only if the signs are clinically severe and not improving after that initial period of time (AHCPR, 1994; Spitzer et al., 1987). The objective of the consultation is to obtain an opinion regarding the need for surgical intervention. Because most neurologic signs resolve without surgery, it is now believed by many consultants that it is best to postpone the consultation until the unremitting nature of the neurologic signs is demonstrated. Only then should one consider further therapeutic options.

The importance of assessing neurologic signs in detail both initially

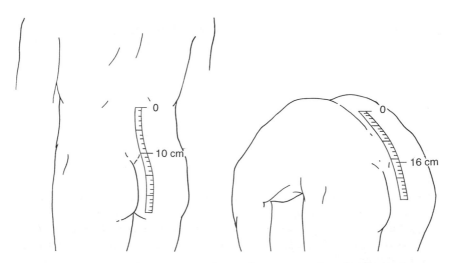

Figure 12–2. The Schober test. The midpoint on a line between the two posterior superior iliac spines is marked. With the patient standing erect, another midpoint line is marked 10 cm above the first line. The patient is asked to bend as far forward as possible and the distance between these points is measured again. In a normal person the distance would increase to be about 16 cm.

and at each visit is not only to make a diagnosis but also to follow the clinical status. Furthermore, it is also very important that the patient understands the nature of the examination that is being performed and the significance of the results in the context of the natural history.

Initial Clinical Diagnosis

At the first visit of a worker with back pain, the description of the pain and the physical examination lead to a diagnosis whose main purpose is to rule out conditions that require urgent intervention (see Table 12–1). In the acute phase, the clinical presentation can be quite dramatic, and the pain can become worse in the first 48 hours than it was when the injury actually occurred. There can be a gradual tightening of the muscles around the injury site, which will contribute to the pain and stiffness. The initial impression is translated into a diagnosis that is written on a compensation system medical certificate. This initial diagnosis has turned out to be a predictor of chronicity, according to research conducted by Abenhaim et al. (1995). The specific diagnoses, mainly sciatica, lesions of the discs, and osteoarthritis, had five times the risk of chronicity as the nonspecific diagnoses (i.e., back pain, sprain, and strain). Four arguments were proposed to explain such a result:

1.   The pathophysiology of lesions with a specific diagnosis leads to a natural history with a poorer prognosis, as previously documented for sciatic pain.

2.   The initial specific diagnosis leads to more investigations and consultations, which potentially delay the therapy and the return to work.

3.   Specific diagnoses such as osteoarthritis can be processed as an occupational disease rather than an injury, and the administrative process to compensate a disease can take more time than for an injury.

4.   Finally, some specialists of the musculoskeletal system have suggested that these results can be explained by a "labeling effect" that would occur between the initial treating physician and the injured worker.

In light of the philosophy underlying the current guidelines for the management of back pain, the fourth argument is interpreted as an emphasis on the diagnostic process that, in the absence of a red flag, is not considered helpful in the first 4 weeks. Indeed, an overemphasis on neurologic signs or a prescription of specialized diagnostic techniques too soon in the clinical management might carry a message of severity to the patient and become a barrier to his or her taking an active part in recovery.

Unlike those for many other medical conditions, the guidelines for management of low back pain recommend delaying diagnostic testing and consultations. There are two reasons for this. First, from what we know of the natural history of back pain, over 80 per cent of the patients recover within 4 weeks of the injury. Therefore, any diagnostic testing before then will not be useful in the majority of the cases. Second, a diagnostic emphasis, in the absence of red flags, through fear of a severe injury may cause the worker to adopt a passive role, which goes against the therapeutic principles for recovery from a back injury. Delaying tests and procedures must be seen within the context of a stepwise diagnostic process that consists of a closely monitored assessment of both physiologic and psychological developments.

FUNCTIONAL STATUS

Pain and physical signs have shown a poor correlation with the functional limitations resulting from back problems (Deyo, 1988). For this reason, there has been much effort devoted to the development of instruments to assess the physical, social, and occupational functioning of individuals with back pain. Table 12–3 summarizes some characteristics of the four most cited instruments and two newer ones. Only the last on the list (the Quebec Back Pain Disability Scale, included in Appendix IV) exclusively focuses on limitations at work. All others explore more or less all the same aspects of pain, activities of daily living, and social life. Some include several constructs of back pain–related disability, such as the Dallas Pain Questionnaire, which includes five different constructs.

Experience acquired with these various instruments clearly shows that the measure of functional status in workers with low back pain is an essential component of the prognosis. Their responsiveness to clinical change allows separation of the functional capacity from the pain component. This is an advantage in the pursuit of functional recovery independent of pain control as a therapeutic goal. Another advantage of these functional scales is that they are all self-administered, and therefore provide feedback to the patients on their own progress.

The *roles of the functional assessment* can be summarized as follows:

1. The responsiveness of the instruments allows follow-up of the changes in back condition more accurately than does asking "How do you feel today?" or "How is your pain today?"

2. The capacity to carry out activities at work and outside the workplace correlates poorly with the pain. The functional assessment is therefore an instrument of prime importance in the evaluation of the capacity to return to work.

3. The functional assessment is useful to determine the limitations that would be applicable for a return to work when there is residual loss of function or pain. In those instances, the functional assessment can also be used to monitor progress following return to work.

4. Because most of the instruments are self-administered, the functional assessment has the advantages of requiring the participation of the injured worker and providing immediate feedback.

RETURN TO WORK/ACTIVITIES

Compensation agencies ask the physician to predict the time of return to work. This is a task that requires planning with the injured worker as early as the initial visit. The health professional must be able to give a prognostic opinion on the capacity to return to work

TABLE 12–3. Instruments Assessing Functional Limitations of Patients with Low Back Pain

INSTRUMENT	SOURCE	NUMBER OF ITEMS/ ANSWERS	VALIDITY	CONTENT	SPECIFICITY OF ACTIVITIES TO WORK	REMARKS
Oswestry Low Back Pain Disability Questionnaire	Fairbank et al. (1980)	10 items, 6-point scale	Reliability Responsiveness Internal consistency	Pain Activities of daily living Social life	No	Widely used and cited in clinical research Item on sex life has poor acceptability
Million questionnaire	Million et al. (1982)	15 items, visual analog scale	Reliability Responsiveness	Pain Activities of daily living Work disability	2 items	Combines constructs of physical impairment and disability
Roland's adaptation of the S.I.P* Questionnaire	Roland and Morris (1983)	24 items, yes/no	Reliability Correlates with pain scale and clinical evaluation	Activities of daily living Psychological impact	No	Correlates differentially between pain and clinical evaluation Adaptation of a widely used scale

Instrument	Reference	Items/Scale	Psychometric properties	Domains		Comments
Waddell questionnaire	Waddell and Main (1984)	9 items, yes/no	Reliability Internal consistency	Activities of daily living Social life	No	Content derived from patients who had a lumbar intervertebral fusion
Dallas Pain Questionnaire	Lawlis et al. (1989)	16 items, visual analog scale	Reliability Internal consistency Discriminates patients with chronic low back pain from normals Correlates with McGill Pain Questionnaire	Pain Activities of daily living Social life Psychological impact Work disability	1 item	Combines 5 different constructs
Quebec Back Pain Disability Scale	Kopec et al. (1995)	a) 20 items, 6-point scale	Reliability Internal consistency	Activities of daily living	No	Only instrument specific to activities at work
		b) 10 items, 4-point scale	Correlates with: pain scale, Roland, Oswestry, SF-36 ph,[+] clinical status, compensation status	At work: physical efforts, posture/movement	Yes	Only instrument to explore the positive aspect of residual capacity

*S.I.P., Sickness Impact Profile.
[+]SF-36 pH: Ware and Sherbourne (1992).

that does not depend solely on the worker's perception of capacity to work. It should also take into consideration the worker's symptomatic and functional state, the occupational history, the task description, and an evaluation by an occupational therapist when needed.

Initial Occupational History

At the first visit, a brief occupational history should be taken to evaluate the stability of the job and the level of specialization of the worker in the past year. Specifically, the questions could enquire about (1) the current type of job and type of industry, and (2) the employment pattern in the past year. This will help determine initially how important the current job is to this individual. For instance, an unskilled worker who has changed jobs several times in the recent past might be less likely to consider the current job as filling a need other than economic. With compensation replacing part of that need, there might be little incentive to return to work, and the physician must be prepared to make a judgment about return to work, independently from the worker's perception.

Job Description

The changes in symptoms and functional ability during the first 4 weeks must be closely followed for any sign of improvement, even temporary. The sawtooth pattern of the natural history of back pain generates expectation that any improvement, even small, will be followed by a bigger one, separated by increase in pain that can be as bad as the initial state. When this pattern is seen, it is important to initiate, at the first sign of improvement, the preparation for a return to work by obtaining a detailed job description. The current evidence suggests that obtaining this description early results in a better prognosis (Lindstrom et al., 1992; Mitchell and Carmen, 1990). A minimal task description would include

the type and frequency of physical effort required
the postures, especially those that must be maintained
the pace
the possibility to do a job in different ways
the amount of standing and walking
environmental factors such as noise, temperature, air pollution, and vibration.

The health care practitioner is not expected to perform a detailed job description, but these six items can help establish the basic parameters for a return to work.

Perception of Incapacity to Work

There can be barriers to a return to work that have little to do with the back problem itself. These barriers are important to identify so that a back injury does not become an argument in the dynamic of a conflict at work. Poor work relations and open conflicts in the workplace can be documented in part by using the "work APGAR," a simple 7-item questionnaire (Bigos et al., 1991) (see Table 12–4).

When planning the return to work, a worker who believes his or her job is not flexible enough to accommodate the residual back pain may be quite correct. However, such a view may be simply a sign of apprehension about aggravating the pain. Such a perception presents a barrier to recovery because it ties pain control and functional recovery into a single therapeutic goal, complete resolution of the pain. If this is suspected, a worker's "avoidance behavior" can be evaluated with the Fear-Avoidance Beliefs Questionnaire, which is specific to low back pain disability (Waddell et al., 1993). This is reproduced in Table 12–5. It consists of 16 items answered on a 7-point scale. A high score might uncover the presence of important psychological problems that are not necessarily related to the return to work itself. The exact nature of such problems might require a referral for psy-

TABLE 12–4.   Modified Work APGAR*

RESPONSE TO QUESTIONS	ALMOST ALWAYS	SOME OF THE TIME	HARDLY EVER
1) I am satisfied that I can turn to a fellow worker for help when something is troubling me.			
2) I am satisfied with the way my fellow workers talk things over with me and share problems with me.			
3) I am satisfied that my fellow workers accept and support my new ideas or thoughts.			
4) I am satisfied with the way my fellow workers respond to my emotions, such as anger, sorrow, or laughter.			
5) I am satisfied with the way my fellow workers and I share time together.			
6) I enjoy the tasks involved in my job.			
7) Please check the column that indicates how well you get along with your closest or immediate supervisor.			

*Reprinted by permission from Bigos SJ, Battie MC, Spengler DM, et al: A prospective study of work perceptions and psychosocial factors affecting the report of back injury. *Spine* 16:1–6, 1991.

TABLE 12–5. Fear-Avoidance Beliefs Questionnaire*

Here are some of the things which other patients have told us about their pain. For each statement please circle any number from 0 to 6 to say how much physical activities such as bending, lifting, walking or driving affect or would affect *your* back pain.

	Completely disagree			Unsure			Completely agree
1. My pain was caused by physical activity	0	1	2	3	4	5	6
2. Physical activity makes my pain worse	0	1	2	3	4	5	6
3. Physical activity might harm my back	0	1	2	3	4	5	6
4. I should not do physical activities which (might) make my pain worse	0	1	2	3	4	5	6
5. I cannot do physical activities which (might) make my pain worse	0	1	2	3	4	5	6

The following statements are about how your normal work affects or would affect your back pain.

	Completely disagree			Unsure			Completely agree
6. My pain was caused by my work or by an accident at work	0	1	2	3	4	5	6
7. My work aggravated my pain	0	1	2	3	4	5	6
8. I have a claim for compensation for my pain	0	1	2	3	4	5	6
9. My work is too heavy for me	0	1	2	3	4	5	6
10. My work makes or would make my pain worse	0	1	2	3	4	5	6
11. My work might harm my back	0	1	2	3	4	5	6
12. I should not do my normal work with my present pain	0	1	2	3	4	5	6
13. I cannot do my normal work with my present pain	0	1	2	3	4	5	6
14. I cannot do my normal work till my pain is treated	0	1	2	3	4	5	6
15. I do not think that I will be back to my normal work within 3 months	0	1	2	3	4	5	6
16. I do not think that I will ever be able to go back to that work	0	1	2	3	4	5	6

Scoring:
Scale 1: fear-avoidance beliefs about work—items 6, 7, 9, 10, 11, 12, 15.
Scale 2: fear-avoidance beliefs about physical activities—items 2, 3, 4, 5.

*Reproduced with permission from Waddell G, Newton M, Henderson I, et al: A Fear-Avoidance Beliefs Questionnaire (FABQ) and the role of fear-avoidance beliefs in chronic low back pain and disability. Pain 52:157–168, 1993.

chological evaluation. Handling this situation will require good skills in interpersonal relationships so that the injured worker does not interpret that course of action as a denial of the back problem.

A worker who has not returned to work after 2 to 3 months and who shows no sign of improvement should be referred to a center offering multidisciplinary care for back problems. Techniques such as work hardening and therapeutic return to work have shown potential benefit in the chronicization and chronic stages (Lindstrom et al., 1992; Mitchell et al., 1990) before chronicity is installed. At the chronicization stage, the role of primary care providers should be to remain in contact with the worker and the multidisciplinary team, in order to ensure continuity of care throughout the current and potential subsequent episodes. The team will generate new information that will become part of the individual's medical history.

Beyond the Return to Work

One follow-up visit should be scheduled soon after the date of return to work, to monitor the pain and functional status as the work activities are being resumed. An increase in pain is expected, especially at the end of the first few working days. The worker should be informed of that and of the risk of recurrences, especially in the first months after the injury. In recurrent episodes, an early diagnosis is the key to prompt and successful recovery.

OTHER PROGNOSTIC ISSUES

Imaging Diagnostic Tests

The Quebec Task Force on activity-related spinal disorders demonstrated the lack of scientific evidence for using any kind of imaging techniques, and some evidence against the use of myelography and discography in the first 7 weeks in the absence of red flags (Spitzer et al., 1987). The AHCPR recommendations are much the same, with a time interval of 4 weeks instead of 7 (AHCPR, 1994). The poor reliability of imaging techniques and their lack of correlation with clinical status (Gibson, 1988) are the reasons why experts do not recommend using them—even plain radiographs, unless to rule out a red flag or to prepare for surgery. With these recommendations, patients' expectations of receiving a radiograph, a computerized tomography scan, or another imaging technique can be met if the limited role of imaging with back pain is explained (Deyo et al., 1987). Individuals with back pain need an explanation for their problem, but this must not be pursued with a quest for an anatomic lesion. It is important to mention here that imaging techniques are often required for compensation or legal purposes. The results of the tests are then interpreted in that context, often ignoring their clinical significance.

A Diagnosis for the Compensation System

Workers' compensation agencies ask physicians to make a diagnosis: initially to confirm that there is a lesion and to validate a claim, and later to authorize the return to work and specify its conditions. Sometimes claim agents can be very insistent, trying to return workers to work as soon as possible. They might have stories concerning a worker who has been seen working around the house while being compensated. The clinician should not be closed to communications with the compensation agents, but should always exert caution in order to preserve confidentiality and avoid becoming prejudiced in the diagnostic and prognostic evaluation. If each worker seen is evaluated in a similar and systematic fashion, emphasizing the elements that have a known prognostic value, as in this chapter, the health care practitioner will be sure to have fulfilled his or her role in a fair manner, independently from other sources of information that the compensation agency collects.

Compensation agencies sometimes will ask a physician to confirm if a back problem is a new episode or a recurrence of a previous one. There are, at the present time, no objective means to make that kind of distinction clinically. The terms are usually defined administratively, using the dates of accidental events. The philosophical and administrative debate regarding this issue is usually deferred to professionals who specialize in giving expert opinions.

Finally, compensation agencies and insurance carriers are often interested in identifying malingerers. The diagnosis of back pain is largely subjective and based on the patient's description. The clinician may assess the validity of the patient's accounts by assessing the degree of collaboration during the clinical exam. As noted in Chapter 9, there are simple tests that have been developed for this purpose (Brown et al., 1954; Waddell and Main, 1984). They are partly based on test-retest reliability assessments. The poor collaboration of a patient, however, is not usually an indication of malingering. It can be related to a psychological condition, or a dissatisfaction with care, that brings the patient to amplify the symptoms. The recognition of such is important for the clinical management but should not be used to label a patient, especially with claim agents. It is generally agreed that true malingerers, who simulate a back problem with the sole objective of getting time off work, are rare. In any case, it is not the role of the health care practitioner to detect malingerers or participate in the investigation of malingering.

REFERENCES

Abenhaim L, Rossignol M, Gobeille D, et al: The prognostic consequences in the making of the initial medical diagnosis of work-related back injuries. Spine 20:791–795, 1995.

Agency for Health Care Policy and Research: Acute Low Back Problems in Adults (Clinical Practice Guideline Number 14) (Publication Number 95-0642). Rockville MD, Agency for Health Care Policy and Research, 1994.

Bigos SJ, Battié MC, Spengler DM, et al: A prospective study of work perceptions and psychosocial factors affecting the report of back injury. Spine 16:1–6, 1991.

Brown T, Nemiah JC, Barr JS, et al: Psychologic factors in low-back pain. N Engl J Med 251:123–128, 1954.

Butler RJ, Johnson WG, Baldwin ML: Managing work disability: Why first return to work is not a measure of success. Ind Labour Relations Rev 48:452–469, 1995.

Deyo RA: Measuring the functional status of patients with low back pain. Arch Phys Med Rehabil 69:1044–1053, 1988.

Deyo RA, Diehl AK, Rosenthal M: How many days of bed rest for acute low back pain? A randomized clinical trial. N Engl J Med 315:1064–1070, 1986.

Deyo RA, Diehl AK, Rosenthal M: Reducing roentgenography use: Can patient expectations be altered? Arch Intern Med 147:141–145, 1987.

Deyo RA, Walsh NE, Martin DC, et al: A controlled trial of transcutaneous electrical nerve stimulation (TENS) and exercise for chronic low back pain. N Engl J Med 322:1627–1634, 1990.

Fairbank JCT, Couper J, Davies JB, O'Brien JP: The Oswestry Low Back Pain Disability Questionnaire. Physiotherapy 66:271–273, 1980.

Gibson ES: The value of preplacement screening radiography of the low back. Occup Med 3:91–107, 1988.

Hadler NM: Regional musculoskeletal diseases of the low back, cumulative trauma versus single incident. Clin Orthop 221:33–41, 1987.

Hirsch C: Reflections on the use of surgery in lumbar disc disease. Orthop Clin North Am 2:493–498, 1971.

Kelsey JL: An epidemiological study of acute herniated lumbar intervertebral discs. Rheumatol Rehabil 14:144–159, 1976.

Kopec JA, Esdaile JM, Abrahamowicz MI: The Quebec Back Pain Disability Scale: Measurement properties. Spine 20:341–352, 1995.

Lawlis GF, Cuencas R, Selby D, et al: The development of the Dallas Pain Questionnaire: An assessment of the impact of spinal pain on behaviour. Spine 14:511–516, 1989.

Lindstrom I, Ohlund C, Eek C, et al: The effect of graded activity on patients with subacute low back pain: A randomized prospective clinical study with an operant-conditioning behavioral approach. Phys Therapy 72:279–293, 1992.

MacRae IF, Wright V: Measurement of back movement. Ann Rheum Dis 28:584–589, 1969.

Malmivaara A, Hakkinen U, Aro T, et al: The treatment of acute low back pain—bed rest, exercises or ordinary activity? N Engl J Med 332:351–355, 1995.

Manning DP, Mitchell DRG, Blanchfield LP: Body movements and events contributing to accidental and nonaccidental back injuries. Spine 9:734–739, 1984.

Mayer TG, Gatchel RJ, Mayer H, et al: A prospective two-year study of functional restoration in industrial low back injury: An objective assessment procedure. JAMA 258:1763–1767, 1987.

Mayo NE, Goldberg MS, Poitras B, et al: The Ste. Justine Adolescent Idiopathic Scoliosis Cohort Study, Part III: Back pain. Spine 19:1573–1581, 1994.

Melzack R, Wall PD: The Challenge of Pain. New York, Basic Books, 1982.

Million R, Hall W, Haavik NK, et al: Assessment of the progress of the back-pain patient. Spine 7:204–212, 1982.

Mitchell RI, Carmen GM: Results of a multicenter trial using an intensive active exercise program for the treatment of acute soft tissue and back injuries. Spine 15:514–521, 1990.

Nachemson AL: Newest knowledge of low back pain: A critical look. Clin Orthop 279:8–20, 1992.

Ransford AO, Cairns D, Mooney V: The pain drawing as an aid to the psychological evaluation of patients with low back pain. Spine 1:127–134, 1976.

Roland M, Morris R: A study of the natural history of back pain. Part I: Development of a reliable and sensitive measure of disability in low back pain. Spine 8:141–144, 1983.

Rossignol M, Suissa S, Abenhaim L: The evolution of compensated occupational spinal injuries: A three-year follow-up study. Spine 17:1041–1047, 1992.

Schober P: Lendenwirbelsaule und Kreuzschmenrzen. Munch Med Wochenschr 84:336–348, 1937.

Spitzer WO, LeBlanc FE, Dupuis M, et al: Scientific approach to the assessment and management of activity-related spinal disorders. Spine 12(Suppl 7):S1–S59, 1987.

Waddell G: A new clinical model for the treatment of low back pain. Spine 12:632–644, 1987.

Waddell G: Biopsychosocial analysis of low back pain. Clin Rheumatol Int Pract Res 6:523–557, 1992.

Waddell G, Main C: Assessment of severity in low back disorders. Spine 9:206–208, 1984.

Waddell G, Newton M, Henderson I, et al: A Fear-Avoidance Beliefs Questionnaire (FABQ) and the role of fear-avoidance beliefs in chronic low back pain and disability. Pain 52:157–168, 1993.

Ware JE, Sherbourne CD: The MOS 36-item short form health survey (SF-36). Med Care 30:473–483, 1992.

Weber H, Holme I, Amlie E: The natural course of acute sciatica with nerve root symptoms in a double-blind placebo-controlled trial evaluating the effect of piroxicam. Spine 18:1433–1438, 1993.

White LA: The evolution of back school programs. Occup Med 7:1–8, 1992.

Yu TS, Roht LH, Wise RA, et al: Low back pain in industry: An old problem revisited. J Occup Med 26:517–524, 1984.

13

Psychological Assessment of Chronic Upper Extremity Disorders

Brad Grunert

A variety of factors are known to influence the experience of physical symptoms (Pennebaker, 1982). In order to appropriately assess the psychological impact of physical symptoms on the individual experiencing them, it is important to identify these factors. Foremost among these is the actual nature of the nociceptive stimulus. The nociceptive stimulus in turn is subject to both an appraisal/evaluative component of perception and an affective/behavioral reaction to it. It is in these areas that the influence of psychological factors is paramount. The entire process of labeling, defining, and describing the nociceptive stimulus as it is experienced by the individual is one that is heavily influenced by personal interpretations and perceptions of reality. This, then, becomes the keystone in the appropriate psychological assessment of individuals experiencing chronic upper extremity disorders.

The nociceptive stimulus has a variety of ways in which it influences the individual. The first of these is the physiologic arousal that is produced as a reaction to a painful or uncomfortable stimulus. Second, a variety of environmental cues and associated learning occur in conjunction with the discomfort that influence future behavior. Additionally, behaviors and emotions result from this learning process that become secondarily conditioned to the experience of the pain and discomfort. Finally, all of these occur within a social context that also has its own rewards and costs for the behavior that occurs secondarily to the discomfort the individual experiences.

Psychological assessment of workers with chronic upper extremity disorders should consist of three basic processes. The first of these is the clinical interview that is conducted with the worker. Second, psychometric assessment is a well-established process that can give further insights into the physical, psychological, and cognitive factors that influence the worker as well as his or her perceptions of the circumstances that are being encountered. Finally, a diagnostic statement must be made that indicates the extent and domains of psychological dysfunction occurring in the worker. When all of these components are in place, a treatment plan can be formulated that will best address the needs of the worker being assessed. (A cognitive-behavioral methodology of treatment is presented in Chapter 16.)

CLINICAL INTERVIEW

History of Onset

In the clinical interview, it is important to first address the history of the perceived onset of symptomatology. The individual frequently attributes various causative factors to the onset of upper extremity difficulties. People tend to emphasize some of these components more than others, and therefore, arrive at psychological models to explain their symptoms. Additionally, they tend to make attributions as to who is responsible for these symptoms. Such attributions heavily influence their adaptation to chronic upper extremity disorder. It is important to assess the nature of the worker's own sense of personal responsibility in the development of symptoms. Those individuals who have worked at a piece-rate job and have consistently overproduced may recognize their own role in the development of cumulative trauma symptoms. Conversely, they may also ascribe the cause of these symptoms to the fact that their employer does not pay them sufficiently and structures the situation so that they need to overproduce in order to make an adequate living. Furthermore, they may also attribute the development of their symptomatology to a variety of environmental factors, most of which can be subsumed under the label of ergonomics. Therefore, these workers may view the environment as being inherently structured to lead them to the development of the symptoms that they are experiencing. This is particularly true if other co-workers also experience symptoms of chronic upper extremity discomfort.

In this situation, the sole responsibility for remediating the situation is assigned to the employer. Often there is a rather hostile interchange between the employee and the employer in this regard. Much like previous research conducted with acute hand injury patients within an industrial setting (Grunert et al, 1988, 1990, 1992), employers may be seen as having breached the basic agreement between the employee and the employer. In its most basic form, this is an agreement that the employee will perform an honest day's work within the restrictions and rules laid out by the employer, and that the employer will provide a safe environment for the employee to do this in. Once this contract is perceived to be broken, there is significant distrust on the part of both the employee and the employer. Often with cumulative trauma disorders, the employer considers the employee to be exaggerating symptoms because there is no visible sign that an injury has occurred. The employer therefore often feels taken advantage of in an unfair manner, and this promotes further hostility.

In addition, factors that are generally overlooked in terms of the history of perceived onset include personal health and health risk factors. There is evidence that people who smoke or are significantly overweight are at higher risk for developing neuropathies and other cumulative trauma disorders of the upper extremity. Additionally, lack of exercise can contribute further to an individual's inability to tolerate the factors that may be leading to the development of a cumulative trauma disorder. As discussed earlier in this book, tissues can be strengthened through long-term use, and this certainly applies to exercise in the context of overall fitness. Most people are very reluctant to examine these factors because there is no clear relationship between their symptomatology and their health risk factors insofar as short-term development of these is concerned. Additionally, workers often believe that, if these factors are examined, the employer is behind the examination as a means of attempting to decline responsibility within the workers' compensation system for the difficulties they are experiencing. Nevertheless, we have found it important within our own hand clinic to work with individuals on lifestyle changes as well as symptoms remediation in order to achieve the best results in treating chronic upper extremity disorders.

Individual Impact of the Problem

The second area that must be focused on in the clinical interview is the impact of the problem on the individual in various ways (Table 13–1). Workers must be questioned extensively about limitations in their own activities and recreation in their daily life. Often these have been the first to be sacrificed as a means of maintaining their employment as well as managing their symptoms. Second, the limita-

TABLE 13–1. Structure of Clinical Interview

History of perceived onset of symptoms
    Personal responsibility versus employer's role
    Personal health factors versus occupational risk factors

Impact of the problem on the individual's
    Personal and recreational activity
    Job performance, peer appraisal
    Perception regarding future health and employability
    Mood (fear, anxiety, depression, anger)
    Family relationships

Coping abilities—stoicism versus somatization

Physiologic factors that have an impact on psychological adjustment
    Sleep disruption
    Depression
    Numbness, tingling
    Weakness, fatigue

tions in the work setting that they perceive to be present are evaluated. It is typically when these work-setting limitations begin to develop that employees become concerned, and begin reporting symptoms and seeking medical care for them. If workers perceive themselves as being unable to accomplish the job that they have been assigned in their work setting, there may be many secondary concomitants, including the possible loss of job, demotion, or the perception by their employers or peers that they are complainers and are unwilling to pull their own weight in the work setting. Additionally, with intervention, the hidden disability often becomes a very visible disability through the application of splints and modifications in the work environment. Once this occurs, the worker is subject to all of the questions, comments, and judgments that arise from the social context of the work setting. These may be either supportive or destructive to the worker.

Affective reactions also must be examined for these individuals. Often they are anxious and concerned that something unknown to them is occurring within their body. Particularly with the bizarre neurologic symptoms that are often experienced in conjunction with the development of cumulative trauma disorders, people become fearful that they are contracting some fatal disease or have a life-threatening condition. Although this does not obtain in a large portion of this population, those in whom it does occur can experience profound emotional disruption. Additionally, even for individuals who understand the condition that they are experiencing, such symptoms are irritating in terms of the consequences that they produce. These workers may have fears and worries over the future of their job, depression resulting from secondary sleep disturbance, and anger or frustration expressed toward the workplace because of their development of symptoms. There may be psychosocial and familial consequences, which again may either support the individual in the expression of his or her symptoms or prove to be costly in terms of loss of ongoing social support. The impact of each of these factors must be assessed in detail in order to arrive at a diagnosis as well as an appropriate treatment plan.

Individual Coping Abilities

A third area that must be assessed in any psychological interview are the coping abilities that the individual has at his or her disposal. In this regard, it is often helpful to examine past health problems and to look at how the worker has coped with these. Some people are very stoic and fail to report symptoms until they are quite progressed. This is often true of the individual who presents to the physician with marked atrophy of the thenar or hypothenar muscles to the point where these are really no longer functioning. Such individuals have experienced symptoms for prolonged periods of time but have basically ignored the symptoms until they were no longer able to function in the manner that was required for their job. In contrast, there are people who are quick to somatize their difficulties and become hypersensitive to any symptomatology that is present. In these individuals, the tiniest of changes are reported as having major consequences for them. They often present to the clinic far before there is any objective documentation for their condition. In such cases, although they may be the individuals who would be most responsive to early intervention, they often have the poorest outcome because they are hypersensitive and hypervigilant to their symptomatology. It is important therefore, to assess the beliefs that shape the meanings of the symptoms for the workers involved.

Physiologic Factors

Physiologic factors also must be assessed in terms of their impact on the psychological adjustment to chronic upper extremity difficulties. It is important to view typical stress reactions and how the worker is coping with these. Each individual has a variety of coping skills, and how these are implemented to handle the ongoing stress of cumulative trauma disorder is particularly important for this population. Additionally, many of these individuals have significantly disrupted sleep, which again results in a whole host of problems.

Because their sleep is more disrupted, they frequently are more easily fatigued and have less energy on the job. Their concentration may not be as good as it was before, putting them at higher risk for other injuries. Depression also frequently accompanies significant and prolonged sleep disruption.

The numbness and tingling, which are a common experience in many of these individuals, often result in feelings of anxiety and irritability. As this progresses, and workers need to shake their arms or hands in the work setting to obtain relief, their difficulties may become more apparent to their peers and, again, the whole social aspect of the work setting can become influential. Weakness is another area which is also of concern for these workers. This is particularly true for piece workers, who may rely a great deal on physical strength and prowess in order to accomplish their job. Because they are not able to keep up production at the same rate, other workers on the line may become irritated and frustrated with them, which may again lead to a variety of social consequences for their symptomatology.

The final factor that is necessary to examine is the experience of pain. Typically, one looks for patterns of descriptors that may indicate the affective loading of the pain for the individual (e.g., "excrutiating, indescribable). The McGill Pain Questionnaire has a full list of such descriptors. Many people experience pain in the work setting and ignore it, whereas others are hypervigilant and report it at the least provocation. All of these factors combine to yield a psychological profile of possible interventions as well as other psychological factors that may be influencing the worker.

PSYCHOMETRIC ASSESSMENT

The second major component of psychological assessment is psychometric assessment (Table 13–2). The *Minnesota Multiphasic Personality Inventory-2*, a test that is very sensitive to individuals who are displaying somatization to an excessive degree, is very useful to administer to all of the individuals who present with chronic upper extremity disorders. There is a classic conversion V that identifies people who tend to sublimate their psychological difficulties under the guise of physical concerns. These individuals find it much easier to address underlying conflicts through effects of physical complaints than they do to address these in a more direct manner psychologically. However, some therapists claim that this personality measure must be used with caution. For example, it is expected that a person

TABLE 13-2. Psychometric Assessment Tools

Minnesota Multiphasic Personality-2 (Hathaway and McKinley, 1989)

Pain Anxiety Symptoms Scale (McCracken et al., 1995)
  Fear
  Cognitive anxiety
  Escape/avoidance
  Physiologic anxiety

Ways of Coping Questionnaire (Folkman and Lazarus, 1988)
  Confrontative coping
  Distancing
  Self-controlling
  Social support
  Accepting responsibility
  Escape/avoidance
  Planful problem solving
  Positive reappraisal

Quality of Life Questionnaire (Evans and Cope, 1980)—15 areas

Occupational Stress Inventory (Osipow and Spokane, 1987)
  Personal strain
  Personal resources
  Occupational role

with an injury will display a higher somatization score as a result of being more physically focused. This does not necessarily imply a hypervigilance to the problem. Therefore, one must interpret a high somatization score with caution. Additionally, this test will yield information on depression, obsessive compulsiveness, and a variety of other psychological conditions.

A second scale that can be administered to workers with chronic upper extremity disorders is the *Pain Anxiety Symptoms Scale*. This scale has four subscales that reveal how individuals react to chronic pain. The first of these is the fear subscale. Basically, this consists of feelings of dread and anxiety that accompany the experience of pain. People who experience high levels of fear in conjunction with the onset of pain typically feel immobilized and have great difficulty in implementing the pain coping strategies that might benefit them. The second scale is cognitive anxiety. When individuals are experiencing cognitive anxiety in reaction to pain, they frequently find it difficult to concentrate and to function adequately in the cognitive sphere. They often become preoccupied with pain and spend a great deal of time thinking about it, which only exacerbates the pain that they experience. The third subscale is the escape/avoidance subscale. Individuals who score high on this subscale, when confronted with pain, typically try to escape or avoid situations in which pain occurs. Again, they tend not to confront their pain and to actively attempt to cope with it, but, rather consistently try to remove themselves from the stimuli that produce the pain for them. The final subscale is the physiologic anxiety scale. On this scale, the individual describes a variety of physiologic reactions to pain. These may include becoming sweaty or having a rapid heart rate. This scale yields a great deal of insight into maladaptive patterns of coping with pain and can have a significant impact on the treatment protocol designed for the worker.

A means of assessing generalized reactions to coping with stress, the *Ways of Coping Questionnaire* consists of eight scales that measure different techniques and strategies for coping with stress. The first of these, the confrontative coping scale, describes aggressive efforts to alter the situation, and a high score suggests that the individual is experiencing some degree of hostility and risk taking. The second scale, the distancing scale, describes efforts to detach oneself and to minimize the significance of the situation. The self-controlling scale reflects efforts to regulate one's feelings and actions. The seeking social support scale describes efforts by the individual to seek support in the social context in order to cope more effectively. The accepting responsibility scale acknowledges that one can have a significant impact on confronting the problem and dealing with it to set the situation right. The escape/avoidance scale describes wishful thinking and behavioral efforts to avoid or escape a problem that are separate from items on the distancing scale, which suggest detachment from the problem. The planful problem solving scale describes deliberate, problem-focused efforts to manage the situation. The final scale, the positive reappraisal scale, describes efforts to create positive meaning by focusing on personal growth. This scale in particular can reveal strengths that can be built on in order to develop an adequate treatment protocol for the worker experiencing ongoing chronic upper extremity discomfort.

A fourth measure, the *Quality of Life Questionnaire*, provides information on 15 different areas of quality of life as well as a general quality-of-life score. Preliminary research that we have conducted with this scale indicates that, in general, individuals experiencing chronic upper extremity disorders have a significantly reduced quality of life in many areas. The areas assessed in the instrument range from material well-being to marital and family relations to political behavior to occupational and job characteristics. In addition, there is a social desirability scale that functions as a validity scale to assess whether persons are attempting to describe themselves in a highly favorable manner.

The final instrument that should be administered on a routine basis is the *Occupational Stress Inventory*. This questionnaire has three domains: the occupational roles questionnaire, the personal strain questionnaire, and the personal resources questionnaire. The occupational roles questionnaire examines the factors of role overload, role insufficiency, role ambiguity, role boundaries, responsibility, and the physical environment. The personal strain questionnaire focuses on vocational strain, psychological strain, interpersonal strain, and physical strain. Finally, the personal resources questionnaire focuses on recreation, self-care, social support, and rational/cognitive coping. This inventory gives significant information regarding each of these areas. When combined with the other instruments described here in an assessment battery, it specifically gives information related to the work setting and how workers view themselves within this.

DIAGNOSTIC STATEMENT

By combining the clinical interview with the psychometric instruments described in the previous section, the clinician can obtain extensive information related to the psychological adjustment of workers experiencing cumulative trauma disorders of the upper extremity. Additionally, the psychometric instruments selected can be used as outcome measures to determine whether or not an individual has progressed over a course of treatment and over time. Administration of these instruments at the time of admission as well as at 6-month and 1-year follow-ups may be quite supportive in identifying those individuals who have benefited from treatment.

The entire process described to this point leads to the issue of differential diagnosis. The primary goal of the assessment is really twofold. The first of these is *to develop an adequate treatment plan* that addresses both the strengths and weaknesses (adaptive and maladaptive responses) of the worker experiencing cumulative trauma disorder. By spelling out psychometrically and through the interview their perceptions of their problem and the strategies that they already have at their disposal for coping, a more personalized program can be developed to assist injured workers in maximizing their adjustment. This is much more effective than a generic approach, which is frequently used in many facilities to address these concerns.

The second major reason for conducting psychological evaluation is *to identify those individuals who have primarily psychological problems* as opposed to physical problems. These would include people with somatoform pain disorders, conversion disorders, factitious disorders, and significant depression that is not the result of chronic pain. Some injured workers can legitimately experience psychological problems such as depression or post-traumatic stress disorders, and require concurrent psychological and physical treatments. Each of these problems consumes vast resources when attempts are made to treat workers in a purely physical context. Furthermore, there is a very low rate of success associated with the treatment of these individuals in such a context. It is important, therefore, to appropriately identify these workers very early in order to structure an appropriate treatment program for them.

Present figures for workers referred to this author's clinic with chronic cumulative trauma disorders reveal that approximately 10 per cent have a primary diagnosis of conversion disorder. Additionally, approximately 3 per cent have diagnoses of factitious disorders. The incidence of somatoform pain disorders is approximately 10 per cent in this population. Slightly less than one quarter of workers referred to this chronic cumulative disorder clinic, therefore, have diagnoses that are primarily psychological rather than physical. Obviously, the treatment plans for such individuals will differ significantly from those of workers who come in with a primarily physical diagnosis but are experiencing some difficulties in coping. These individuals also raise a variety of issues related to the workers' compensation system and whether or not it is responsible for funding treatment. There is no question that they are experiencing high levels of discomfort and symptomatology; however, they also fail to respond to traditional treatment programs in any manner. In fact, such programs may be viewed as threatening to them because they are using their physical concerns as a means of obtaining psychological support. Grunert et al. (1991) have discussed some of the diagnostic procedures and management techniques that they have developed for this population.

CONCLUSION

Psychological assessment occupies a key role in the work-up of the individual with chronic cumulative trauma disorder. These individuals often have experienced widespread lifestyle changes as well as significant emotional consequences from their ongoing disability. As a result, an evaluation of the difficulties they are encountering as well as the strengths they have at their disposal for more effective coping is paramount. Additionally, the identification of individuals who are experiencing psychological conditions that will prohibit or severely limit their success in the physically oriented treatment program is also a key concern. Through the identification of specific needs of workers, more appropriate treatment planning can proceed, with greatly enhanced outcomes as a benefit.

REFERENCES

Evans DR, Cope WE: Quality of Life Questionnaire. North Tonawanda, NY, Multi-Health Systems, Inc, 1989.

Folkman S, Lazarus RS: Ways of Coping Questionnaire. Palo Alto, CA, Mind Garden, 1988.

Grunert BK, Devine CA, Matloub HS, et al: Psychological adjustment following work-related hand trauma: 18-month followup. Ann Plast Surg 29: 482–489, 1992.

Grunert BK, Matloub HS, Sanger JR, et al: Treatment of post-traumatic stress disorder after work-related hand trauma. J Hand Surg 15A:511–515, 1990.

Grunert BK, Sander JR, Yousif NJ, et al: A classification system for factitious hand syndromes with implications for treatment. J Hand Surg 16A:1027–1030, 1991.

Grunert BK, Smith CJ, Devine CA, et al: Early psychological aspects of traumatic hand injury. J Hand Surg 13B:177–180, 1988.

Hathaway SR, McKinley JC: Minnesota Multiphasic Personality Inventory-2. Minneapolis, National Computer Systems, 1989.

McCracken LM, Zayfert C, Gross RT: The Pain Anxiety Symptoms Scale (PASS): A multimodal measure of pain specific anxiety symptoms. Behav Ther 16:183–184, 1995.

Osipow SH, Spokane AR: Occupational Stress Inventory. Odessa, FL, Psychological Assessment Resources, Inc, 1987.

Pennebaker JW: The Psychology of Physical Symptoms. New York, Springer-Verlag, 1982.

MANAGEMENT ___

14

Workplace Management of the Injured Worker

Alberta Piché

The nursing management approach presented in this chapter is based on the health promotion model commonly applied in treatment of cardiovascular disease, but adapted to the workplace setting. Such a model focuses on primary, secondary, and tertiary prevention.

Musculoskeletal disorders are generally underreported in the workplace. Therefore, the available prevalence and incidence data probably underestimate their true magnitude. Difficulties and inconsistencies in diagnosis compound this problem. Musculoskeletal disorders are widespread, and although they are not fatal, these disorders account for much disability, pain, and suffering. Accordingly, from productivity losses on the factory floor to medical expenses and compensation for the injured, the cost of workers stricken by musculoskeletal injuries is taking a substantial bite out of the bottom line for many employers.

The key to future success in health care management of the musculoskeletally injured worker at the worksite is the appropriate application of a variety of intervention practices. The occupational health nurse is trained and strategically located to play a vital role in the design and implementation of such interventions. These include accurate diagnosis of the problem, correct medical treatment and worker reassignment, job site accommodation, safe work practice education, progressive transitional work programs, and ergonomically sound job modification. All of these assist the worker to continue at work. If the worker remains employed, then the social and economic burden to the employer and to society as a whole can be reduced over time.

COSTS TO INDUSTRY

Evidence from the United States suggests a slow but steady increase in incidence of musculoskeletal injuries over the last few decades. U.S. Occupational Safety and Health Administration figures show that more than one third of all workers' compensation costs are related to cumulative trauma disorders. A single cumulative trauma disorder injury can cost $30,000 (U.S.) in compensation for medical bills alone. The number of work-related injuries attributable to cumulative trauma disorders in the United States has climbed to 302,000 reported cases in 1993, an increase of more than 7 per cent over the previous year and up 63 per cent from 1990.

The Canadian province of British Columbia is pursuing an ergonomics standard. This is in part because the Canadian Workers' Compensation Board paid out more than $400 million between 1988 and 1992 for more than 100,000 ergonomic-related claims. However, in Canada as a whole, the overall trend in workers' compensation claims has been a gradual decrease over time. This decrease may be attributed to deteriorating labor market conditions, to underreporting of these types of injuries, to a lack of specific diagnosis, or to a combination of these.

It is not critical injuries that account for the bulk of the Canadian compensation case load. Rather, in 1993, sprains and strains made up 42 per cent of work-related injuries and illnesses in Canada, and 53 per cent in 1994. This shows a marked increase of over 38 per cent since 1970 (Globe and Mail, Thursday, April 28, 1996). The Ontario workers' compensation system has some 5,500 chronic pain cases that are reported to have cost Ontario $330 million. In Canada as a whole, according to a Toronto newspaper report, fewer workers are getting hurt on the job. But the cost of their injuries is ballooning—to at least $10 billion annually at last count. One of the primary factors in the cost increase is that injuries have become more chronic and crippling (Globe and Mail, Thursday, April 28, 1996). Untangling the cause of such injuries through analysis of statistics can be very difficult.

ROLE OF THE OCCUPATIONAL
HEALTH NURSE

Nurses working in an occupational setting are well recognized as being, in many cases, the initial primary caregivers for health problems arising at work. Some of these problems are work-related chronic musculoskeletal injuries. However, nurses do not just treat these injuries. Through a combination of special training, location of employment, and on-the-job experience, they also play a key role in prevention of injury. This includes worker and even employer education, identification of unhealthy work practices, and recommendation of measures that will result in a healthier working environment. In this way, their work has foreshadowed the new age in medical management wherein illness prevention will one day supercede illness treatment in relevance.

When a worker is injured, the occupational health nurse faces the challenge of establishing a correct diagnosis so that appropriate treatment can be given and medical referral be made when indicated. However, another vital role in postinjury treatment is the prevention of long-term disability by early and appropriate recommendation of work modification, together with supervision of its implementation and monitoring of the results.

Once a serious overuse injury has been sustained, there is only a limited chance that medical intervention will help to obtain a full recovery. This is the reason both prevention and rehabilitation must be considered together. Primary prevention involves identifying high-risk jobs and preventing musculoskeletal injuries from occurring in the workplace. Secondary prevention of musculoskeletal injuries is the reduction of the extent of disability after an injury has occurred. This involves the development of strategies to allow an injured worker to remain at work without further risk of injury. Tertiary prevention is management in the postrecovery period. However, in practice, there is considerable overlap between these three areas. A preventative program, by its very nature, is required to be comprehensive because it addresses the potential hazards and existing conditions particular to that workplace. Supervisors, management, and labor should be aware from the outset that there is not just one simple solution to a complex problem.

PRIMARY PREVENTION IN THE WORKPLACE

Identification of High-Risk Jobs

The identification of high-risk jobs is the first step in the prevention of work-related injuries. Evaluation of first aid and supervisor accident investigation reports helps determine the total number of musculoskeletal injury cases that are reported. The date each case was reported and the department (or specific process/job) of the workers must be recorded. Then the number of workers on that specific job in the at-risk department must be determined. This information is used to calculate the incidence rate (i.e., the number of new musculoskeletal injuries per department or job for a specific time period) in order to compare with other jobs or departments within the same organization.

Next the occupational health nurse should review available medical and safety records to identify current cases, and then extend the project to include a symptom survey for all employees. This can assist the occupational health nurse to develop a department's risk profile.

Job Analysis

The development of a departmental risk profile also requires job analysis for each of those jobs that are associated with frequent injuries. Such an analysis evaluates work methods, design of workstations, equipment, tools, and work organization in relation to the size, speed, and strength capabilities of the worker's body. It also breaks the job up into a series of tasks that are examined from an ergonomic point of view, as described in Chapter 4.

A job analysis may be job oriented or worker oriented. For the frequently reinjured worker, the job-oriented analysis method is the one of choice. Following injury, in the area of secondary prevention, a job analysis is required to see whether an alternative job can be done by the injured worker.[1] In primary prevention, its purpose is to determine why certain jobs seem more hazardous than others. The job-oriented analysis method will identify tasks of a specific job and determine functional demands placed on an employee by the tasks and by the environment. Each work task is an identifiable work activity that constitutes one of the logical and necessary steps to perform a job (e.g., coding data, preparing technical reports).

The job analyst must establish the exact mechanics of the work performed. To do this, the following information should be obtained:

Job description/qualification (see form in Appendix V)
Physical demands analysis
Exact mechanics of the work performed
Frequency of repetitive motion/cycle time
Whether one hand is used more than the other while working
Whether vibrating or rotary tools are used

---

[1] A job analysis as part of the secondary prevention process will also assist the occupational health nurse in educating the supervisor on how to effectively investigate a musculoskeletal injury in order to detect problems in production work tasks. Solutions to resolve the issue can then be recommended to management and to the health and safety committee of the company.

Length of time performing the particular job

Whether there was a change in work just prior to the onset of symptoms

The worker's production rate per hour or shift in comparison to co-workers performing the same duties

Although not part of the job analysis itself, it is important to know whether the worker's activities outside of work involve any of the recognized risk factors of the job.

The goal is to reduce or eliminate the six generic risk factors for occupational musculoskeletal disorders: rapid or repetitive movements, forceful exertions, external mechanical force concentrations, awkward or "non-neutral" postures, vibration, and cold temperature. In high-risk jobs, often two or more of these factors are present and exert a synergistic adverse effect. Control measures, to be effective, usually need to address all existing exposures. Then the work process in any setting can be redesigned to fit the task to the worker in the most healthful and cost-effective way. An "ergonomic assessment form" used to identify risk factors in the meat processing industry, included in Appendix V, may be found useful in identifying work environment and individual factors.

Employee Health Promotion

Each worker must be trained correctly in the performance of the job, to do it in a manner that is as biomechanically efficient as possible. The usual education about safe work practices, use of personal safety equipment, and which tools to use and how to use them safely is important in preventing acute injuries. However, poor body mechanics, assuming awkward body postures, and working without adequate rest pauses can lead to chronic problems further on in time. Workers must be educated about these matters, be taught and given time to do stretching and strengthening programs, be advised against doing piecework and overtime, and be encouraged to adopt an active lifestyle outside of work. The latter includes good nutrition. Employers need to be educated themselves and be seen to support the educational program.

SECONDARY PREVENTION IN THE WORKPLACE

When the worker presents to the health office, it is apparent that primary prevention has become ineffective and the worker is looking for medical help. Health care providers should be trained in the appropriate interview and clinical examination procedures to diagnose occupational musculoskeletal disorders, as described in earlier chapters of this book. Exposed workers and their supervisors should be informed of the signs and symptoms associated with these conditions as part of the educational program, in order that treatment will be sought earlier. The workers must be taken seriously and referred to appropriate health care practitioners when symptoms persist.

A rehabilitation program is geared to keeping injured workers at work if possible, and, if not, then ensuring that the worker returns to a suitable job as early as possible. The likelihood of achieving success is dependent on the duration of the problem. Chronic musculoskeletal injuries are the result of cumulative trauma. They result from performing repetitive and stressful work elements over extended periods of time. The occupational health nurse should assess the worker and obtain a detailed work history to determine the nature and severity of the disorder, as indicated in Tables 14–1 and 14–2. (The examination techniques are found in Chapters 9, 10, and 11.) Once the problem is identified, there should be no delay in implementing the treatment program.

Treatment

The best treatment for cumulative trauma disorders, according to Weeks et al. (1991), is rest for the affected tendon, joint, or nerve. This

TABLE 14–1.   **Clinical Information That May Be Gathered Regarding the Worker**

Name, age, sex
Body mass index
Number of years employed in present job position
Personal health history: of special significance is the presence of
    rheumatoid arthritis, collagen diseases such as lupus erythematosus,
    other connective tissue disorders, hypertension, diabetes, thyroid
    disorders, gout, kidney disease, and current pregnancy
Medication list
Recent absences from work resulting from injury/illness
Documented past medical history
Occupational history
Documentation of wrist size in case a splint is needed
Physical examination, inspection for signs of inflammation (redness,
    swelling), ganglion cysts, or deformities; palpation for tenderness;
    assessment of active range of motion. Various diagnostic maneuvers
    would include Tinel's test of the median and ulnar nerves. Phalen's test,
    and Finkelstein's test.

TABLE 14–2. Types of Questions To Ask Concerning the Worker's Pain

1. Where is the pain? Use a body diagram (as in Appendix II) to outline the exact location of the pain. If there is more than one pain, mark each separately.
2. When did it begin?
3. How often does it occur?
4. How long does it usually last?
5. What makes it worse?
6. What relieves it?
7. What does it feel like (e.g., sharp, dull, achy, burning, throbbing)?
8. How severe is it? Use a 10-point scale where 0 = no pain and 10 = worst pain imaginable.
9. Has the pain affected activities unrelated to work (e.g., hobbies, recreation)?
10. Along with the pain, are there any other symptoms (e.g., tingling, numbness, stiffness, cramps, spasms)?
11. Have there been sleep problems or emotional upset?

includes rest from work, all household duties, and other manual activities. Rest is sometimes combined with cold compresses for temporary pain relief, anti-inflammatory medication, physical or occupational therapy, or use of splints. However, none of these treatments is likely to be effective if the individual continues to work without appropriate ergonomic modification of the workstation, tools, equipment, and/or workplace.

Splint use on the job should be considered when appropriate, but only if it does not interfere with work or require the worker to exert force or strain on another body part in order to perform the task. A splint is helpful to rest an inflamed tendon if friction is the problem (e.g., de Quervain's tenosynovitis). However, care must be taken that there is no direct pressure on the tendon itself, because this will increase friction if even a small amount of movement is allowed. Splints that are so useful at night for carpal tunnel syndrome have been shown to actually increase hydrostatic pressure within the carpal tunnel when used at work. Therefore, the use of a splint for carpal tunnel syndrome at work is contraindicated.

The treatment protocol is outlined in Table 14–3. It is this author's experience that injuries of short duration usually resolve within 7 to 10 days if such medical management is strictly adhered to. However, injuries of long duration are resistant to treatment, and all the listed methods may already have been tried with no resolution of the problem. It is then that the nurse will need to advise supervisors and others that the only defense against permanent impairment may be removal of the employee from physical or strenuous work, reduction of work hours, and/or assignment to modified/alternate work as the

TABLE 14–3.   Treatment Protocol

1. *Pain treatment*: Nonsteroidal anti-inflammatory medication as medically directed
2. *Cold treatment*: ice wrap applied to area for 15 minutes three to four times per day. Cryotherapy (direct ice application to the skin) may be used for deep tissue cooling if not contraindicated (maximum 2 minutes).
3. Re-evaluate in 2 days and, if symptoms are not improved, then refer to physician, review job description, and recommend corrective changes.
4. Noninvasive pain relief techniques (e.g., relaxation, massage) are applicable unless there is swelling, crepitus, or numbness.
5. Transfer the affected worker to temporary suitable work that has no risk factors.
6. Apply wrist splint only for tenosynovitis and if no wrist bending is required on the job.
7. Re-evaluate in 2 days and, if symptoms have not resolved, continue with temporary suitable work and arrange for medical assessment.
8. Advise a work rehabilitation program that is medically validated and monitored for 6 to 8 weeks; this may need to be extended a further 2 to 4 weeks if medically advised.

situation demands. Initially, the worker's symptoms may disappear with cessation of work, only to recur after the worker resumes work. If the injury gets worse, however, pain may continue even when work ceases. The longer a person works with pain on the same job, the slower the recovery and the greater the risk of permanent harm.

A diagnosis-based treatment program carried out at the worksite enables the injured worker to continue to work within a monitored environment. The occupational health nurse can effect organizational change and support the injured worker in the workplace by helping to remove barriers—for example

Assisting workers to seek a medical opinion about their problem

Safeguarding the affected workers by informing appropriate authorities that being allowed adequate recuperation time away from work is necessary for recovery

Reassigning affected workers to suitable work when they have a permanent disability

Along with physical or drug therapy or both as determined by medical authorities, such methods of treatment are usually effective. However, with a repeated musculoskeletal injury, success may be elusive and require a considerable amount of time and patience. Reasons for failure of treatment in such cases may be psychological, sociological, or related to work organization. These issues are discussed further in Chapter 17.

Process of Planning Accommodations at the Worksite

For the injured worker to be eligible for a modified/alternate work program, the occupational health nurse should: (1) ensure that medical assessment of the injured worker is completed if the symptoms are unresolved; (2) following this, conduct a job analysis as described for primary prevention; (3) determine the functional potential of the worker; (4) compare job analysis data and functional potential of that worker; and (5) identify and evaluate remedial alternatives. The following documentation is required:

A complete medical assessment of the injured worker

A completed physical demands analysis, reviewed by all parties (i.e., family doctor, worker, union, supervisor) and signed by supervisor and worker

A signed release of medical information from the worker

A letter of explanation to the doctor explaining the program goals and objectives

Establishment of the program duration (this depends on the type of injury and should have a limit of no more than 10 weeks)

A completed doctor's report containing a specific diagnosis, functional limitations, duration of the medical precautions, and estimated date to return to regular work (this should be returned by the employee to the supervisor)

Follow-up is important to ensure that job modifications have been effective, that modified/alternate jobs have been correctly selected to avoid continuing stress on the affected part, and that symptoms and signs do not progress further, causing permanent damage.

A work rehabilitation program that is composed of a variety of job choices provides the means for the occupational health nurse to customize the worker's rehabilitation program. This is fundamental for the success of the worker's recovery. Important elements to include in the worker's work rehabilitation program are having available the services of a physiotherapist at the worksite, actual work simulation at the worker's job site or an alternate job site, job rotation, frequent rest/stretch breaks, or job modification. The health care professional can choose from these options to individualize the rehabilitation to the specific worker in the specific job.

TERTIARY PREVENTION

Unfortunately, workers with repeated musculoskeletal injuries continue to work at their regular jobs until the effects of the disability interfere with production demands or activities of daily living. Often these workers will not be able to return to their original jobs. Hence employers would be wise to initiate vocational rehabilitation as early as possible. This involves determining the worker's skills and trainability for the job opportunities available. (See Appendix V for examples of a skill/vocational requirement form and a physical demands analysis form that may be used.)

If the worker has not returned to the regular job and seems likely to exceed the modified work program duration (usually 8 to 10 weeks), it is advisable then to recommend that an ergonomist come on site and do a job analysis. The purpose of this job site or "worksite" analysis is to define the specifics of the job as it relates to the particular chronic injury and to suggest feasible solutions. A preliminary evaluation by the occupational health nurse to identify suspected risk factors should precede the ergonomist's analysis because this saves time and reduces outside costs. Delaying the ergonomist's assessment may lead to decreased employee motivation to continue with the program. This step is critical in the problem-solving process because of the severity and nature of the medical problem.

Further steps to be taken by the occupational health nurse at this time include the following:

1.   Providing education on workplace modifications that prevent musculoskeletal injuries to human resources personnel, health and safety committee members, management, union, and supervisors. A participatory approach is necessary to effect workplace changes. Both labor and management must agree on and endorse these changes.

2.   Assisting the company's health and safety committee to investigate all musculoskeletal injury causes and recommend remedial solutions. One of these may be the creation of an ergonomics committee.

3.   Preparing a list of potentially suitable alternative employment prospects. All too often the occupational health nurse comes face to face with an employer forming premature decisions concerning the worker's employment status, and this usually results in costly mistakes. The nurse can help the employer avoid traversing the legal maze that could be necessary in the eventuality that the injured worker cannot be placed back with the same organization. For this purpose, a hierarchy of employment objectives will prove useful.

The hierarchy of employment objectives describes all the possible vocational outcomes in order of preference. The ideal outcome for an injured worker is to return to the same job with the same employer. Unfortunately, this often may be impossible. At the other end of the spectrum, if a worker must be trained to do an entirely different job for a different employer, the cost in Canada can be as high as $289,000 per worker. A sample hierarchy of employment objectives for an injured worker is as follows:

Objective 1	The client returns to the same job with the same employer without modification of job duties
Objective 2	The client returns to the same job with the same employer but with modifications in job duties
Objective 3	The client returns to the same employer but in a different job that does not require the employer to modify the job duties or the client to receive formal retraining; the worker maintains or approximates previous earning capacity
Objective 4	The client returns to the same employer but in a different job; formal retraining is unnecessary but job duty modifications are required; earning capacity is maintained at the predisability level
Objective 5	The client returns to employment with a different employer performing a similar type of job with or without duty modifications; earning capacity is maintained at the predisability level
Objective 6	The client returns to employment with a different employer at a different job, with or without duty modifications—a job that can be done without formal retraining
Objective 7	The client returns to employment, with the same or a different employer, at a different job only after formal training has been successfully completed
Objective 8	Self-employment

Surgical Rehabilitation Management

Apart from carpal tunnel syndrome, chronic work-related musculoskeletal injuries rarely require surgical intervention. New techniques of endoscopic surgery for carpal tunnel syndrome repair usually have the patient in a wrist splint for about 1 week after surgery. This is to promote healing and prevent median nerve entrapment during wrist flexion. After the second week, the splint and sutures are removed, and patients who do not perform heavy lifting in their jobs are allowed to return to work without restrictions. Patients with heavy lifting jobs usually do not return to unrestricted work until the third week. This technique is currently under review, and time will tell whether it will be generally adopted in place of conventional surgery, which has a longer rehabilitation period.

However, surgery may be only temporarily effective if the worker is returned to an ergonomically stressful job that has not been modified. Use of transitional work programs and gradual introduction back into the work tasks is essential for success. The transitional work program for affected workers, and graded retraining, should be accomplished under the supervision of an experienced physical/occupational therapist or other experienced occupational health care practitioner located at the workplace.

Case Analysis

An overview of prevention strategies, presented in Table 14–4, includes the above topics under the heading of tertiary prevention. It also mentions the case analysis process, which may be applied if other strategies fail and all jobs with the original employer are be-

---

TABLE 14–4. Overview of Prevention in the Workplace

PRIMARY: DECREASING RISK OF INJURY
Identification of high-risk jobs from statistical data
Identification of currently injured cases
Employee symptom survey
Analysis of high-risk job for risk factors
Recommendations to management for work redesign
Employee health promotion
    Training and education
    Job rotation (structured to use different muscle groups)
    Stretch/strengthening exercise programs
    Adequate work/rest cycles
    Elimination of piecework and overtime
    Promotion of active lifestyle programs

SECONDARY: EARLY INTERVENTION IN INJURY EVENTS
Clinical assessment/personal attributes
Assisting injured worker with treatment choices that are available
Assessment of workstation for risk factors so as to reduce or eliminate
    them
Planning of accommodations (this involves job analysis of current and
    possibly alternative work, and finding a job that matches the functional
    capacity of the injured worker)
Identification of barriers to recovery
Development of modified work programs, including transitional work
    programs
Application of hierarchy of employment objectives 1 and 2

TERTIARY: REHABILITATION DURING THE RECOVERY PERIOD
Restoration of worker to highest possible level of preinjury function
Postoperative management where surgery is needed, including transitional
    work programs
Application of of hierarchy of employment objectives 3 through 8
Case analysis process if vocational placement elsewhere is required
Outcome evaluation regarding:
    Expected decline in injury statistics
    Cost effectiveness: on site versus off site
    Consumer satisfaction
    Employability of injured worker

---

yond the capabilities of the injured worker. Discussion of this process relates to disability management, which is beyond the scope of this book. For valuable information on this topic, the reader is referred to Shrey and Lacerte (1995).

CONCLUSION

Occupational health nurses are the gatekeepers to the workplace health care system and strive to maintain the worker's health within a holistic model of prevention and management. In North America, we do not have a healthy health care system, and there are those who believe we do not have a healthy society in general. Often the way the health care system is wounded is the way all of society is wounded. Employers would be wise to view their workers not as economic units but as people with souls, and to listen to them with a new understanding related as much to the spiritual world as to the material world.

REFERENCES

Shrey D, Lacerte M (eds): Principles and Practices of Disability Management in Industry. Winter Park, FL, GR Press Inc, 1995.
Weeks JL, Levy BS, Wagner ER: Preventing Occupational Disease and Injury. Washington, DC, American Public Health Association, 1991.

RECOMMENDED READING

Auleciems L: Myofascial pain syndrome: A multidisciplinary approach. Nurse Pract 20(4):18, 1994.
Hales R, Bertsche P: Management of upper extremity cumulative trauma disorders. Am Assoc Occup Health Nurs J 40(3):118, 1992.
Hall H, McIntosh G, Melles T: Recognition and management of the chronic pain syndrome. Can J CME 7(3):39–49, 1995.
Lacerte M, Wright G: Return to work determination. Phys Med Rehab 6:283, 1992.
Piché A: Case management of the injured worker. J Ontario Occup Health Nurses Assoc 13(2):18, 1994.
Putz-Anderson V: Cumulative Trauma Disorders: A Manual for Musculo-skeletal Diseases of the Upper Limbs. London, Taylor & Francis, 1988.
Rogers, B: Occupational Health Nursing Concepts and Practice. Philadelphia, WB Saunders Company, 1994.

Rogers B, Mastroianni K, Randolph S: Occupational Health Nursing Guidelines for Primary Clinical Conditions. Boston, Occupational and Environmental Medicine Press, 1992.

Travers P: Implementing ergonomic strategies in the workplace: An occupational health nursing perspective. Am Assoc Occup Health Nurs J 40(3): 129, 1992.

15
Physical Therapy for Physical Problems

John Chong

As the number of prescriptions for time off work and for medications rises, so do the enormous associated disability costs. As discussed in the previous chapters, work-related injuries, whether they are called cumulative trauma disorders, repetitive strain injuries, or work-related musculoskeletal disorders, have become the number one occupational health problem. Disability costs have risen astronomically in the past decade. So why not just prescribe rest and anti-inflammatories? The simple answer to this question is the topic of this chapter.

Numerous authors have claimed this medical and societal phenomenon to be a cruel hoax of the greedy medical professional, creating an imaginary illness in compensation-hungry workers. An alternative explanation lies in poor engineering of industrial processes, faulty occupational ergonomics, and the lack of accurate diagnosis and effective treatment for these types of injuries.

The purpose of this chapter is to integrate key concepts in ergonomics and pathophysiology of these injuries. It provides an approach for clinicians who have the responsibility of providing diagnostic and treatment services with the goal of enabling injured workers to return to gainful employment.

DEFINING THE PROBLEM

Problem Analysis: Why Can't This Worker Do This Occupational Task?

The first challenge for the clinician is to understand the worker's occupational functional limitations. By the time medical help is sought, these limitations are often perceived by a worker as a complete inability to perform the job in question. The physical reasons are often reported by a worker as pain in the affected upper extremity, neck, and shoulders, vaguely distributed numbness, and/or difficulty in specific movements required to carry out a task. The clinician must interpret these symptoms in a more sophisticated manner and analyze the problems at the man-machine interface. All too often, intervention is directed only at symptom complaints.

The first step is to take a detailed occupational history. Many types of questionnaires have been used to accomplish this task. A clinically useful questionnaire is provided in Appendix II. Completing the occupational history for each job that the injured worker has undertaken during his or her career is often a laborious task but is crucial to understanding the development of a work-related musculoskeletal disorder. For example, in the contemporary workplace, many individuals carry out a wide variety of occupational tasks that involve repetitive movement and static loading while using microcomputers and customized devices required for specialized production. Occasionally there are more demanding tasks, such as lifting and transporting heavy objects associated with awkward postures. The clinician must understand *all* tasks performed by the worker in order to formulate a clinical hypothesis of the site and severity of injury. This understanding applies equally to *leisure and domestic tasks* that may directly or indirectly be related to the occupational difficulty.

With this background information, the clinician is then in a position to carry out a detailed interview of the injured worker, probing for specific explanations regarding the functional limitations at work. During this interview, it is extremely useful to ask the individual to demonstrate the difficulty so as to minimize the potential for misunderstanding the problem by relying merely on verbal descriptions. For example, a musician can play an instrument and select a specific passage to demonstrate to the clinician the occupational difficulty. In a similar way, a computer operator can show the clinician where the functional problem arises and how this comes about through demonstration rather than description.

The feasibility of demonstration in the clinical setting will obviously decrease if one is dealing with larger equipment such as vibratory tools or manufacturing devices. In this case, it is extremely useful for the clinician to either visit the plant or invite the injured worker or employer to provide videotapes of the task and of the worker performing it. Not all clinicians will have the expertise to make such an analysis, but instructional short courses are available (e.g., through the Faculty of Applied Health Sciences, University of Waterloo, Waterloo, Ontario).

At a very minimum, the worker must be asked during an office interview to demonstrate how the task is performed. Then, with reference to the task analysis methodology given in Chapter 4, decisions can be made about posture and movements that seem to be causally related to the occupational difficulty (see Tables 4–2 through 4–6 in this regard). At this stage, the clinician is now prepared to embark on a problem-solving approach to the analysis and treatment of the work-related musculoskeletal disorder.

Inflammation Analysis: What Is Causing the Worker's Pain?

A problem-oriented physical examination is crucial for the accurate diagnosis and prescription of treatment. The use of a self-administered pain diagram (Appendix II) for patients to complete prior to the examination assists the examiner in localizing areas for careful inspection and palpation. Associated symptoms such as pain, numbness, and other activity-related factors add specific information for the examiner to evaluate.

Techniques of physical examination have been described in Chapters 9, 10, and 11. Forms for recording results are found in Appendix III. In addition, careful observation of *posture and breathing patterns* is crucial for the understanding the pain and functional limitations. Palpation of trigger points and pain referral patterns are well described in the textbook by Travell and Simons (1992), and these techniques should be employed. Examination of proximal musculature of scapular stabilization and cervical support must not be overlooked. This is often neglected in patients who have peripheral symptoms; for example, palpation of the scalene and related cervical muscles, teres minor, or pectoralis minor can often reproduce peripheral symptoms. Examination of the neurovascular bundle for irritation and impingement must be carefully carried out.

During this phase, the examiner attempts not only to reproduce the symptoms but also to understand the relationship of the pain to the causative or aggravating work activity. Only then can the examiner formulate the problem in such a way as to prescribe an effective treatment plan. It is often useful to ask the injured worker to carry out the specific task repetitively before coming for examination in order to bring on the symptoms and signs of the musculoskeletal disorder.

Activity Analysis: What Can This Worker Really Do?

A worker's functional capacity can be determined in a number of ways, from the examination to more formal testing. Flexibility and strength testing are often used to derive conclusions about functional capacity. However, this approach has limited value for tasks that feature highly complex movement patterns or are repetitive over a long duration. The examiner can ask the worker to carry out the task in the clinical setting for a specified duration and examine the change over time. Often this functional assessment is more useful in understanding the nature of the injury and the degree of functional impairment than it is for indicating what the injured worker can do. Such information is also useful in choosing appropriate work in relation to the hierarchy of objectives described in Chapter 14.

Mechanisms of the various musculoskeletal disorders are described in Chapter 3, including the often-overlooked deconditioned muscle. Only after repetitively carrying out the task in a work simulation can this fatigue factor be observed. Once again, a video ergonomic analysis is extremely useful. The suspected site of injury can be surveyed repeatedly with video replay. Often the movement or posture pattern will change over time, and this can be documented objectively. This part of the assessment may be used as a baseline on which clinical progress comparisons may be made at any time. It also serves as an objective record of the functional impairment that may be useful in further diagnostic testing. In a clinic setting, this videotape record can be used to communicate the nature of the functional problem to other members of the therapy team, so that all have a deeper understanding of the problem.

Neurologic Analysis

Because peripheral nerve impingement is common in patients presenting with work-related musculoskeletal disorders, a *thorough examination of the peripheral nerves* is mandatory. Careful assessment of the median, ulnar, and radial nerves and their associated musculature, as described in Chapter 11, is necessary to formulate an appropriate treatment regimen and should be repeated later to assess the response to therapy. There may be early clinical signs of denervation, or intermittent symptoms may be reproduced by specific provocative tests. Static postural problems and dynamic muscle imbalances with repetitive movement can induce regional fatigue and pain. All of these considerations must be borne in mind during clinical assessment.

Electrodiagnostic tests yield clinical information relevant to the functional impairment. Standard nerve conduction velocity tests of sensory and motor nerves and, if necessary, electromyography (EMG) should be carried out by appropriate medical consultants. For monitoring of therapeutic progress, repeat electrodiagnostic tests may sometimes be helpful.

More recently, surface EMG technology has become available for monitoring treatment progress as well as initial functional evaluation. This involves the frequency analysis of the power spectrum of muscle groups required in certain repetitive tasks. Clinical protocols for measurement have been generated that can prove extremely useful, especially for monitoring the fatigue component of the musculoskeletal disorder (Skubick et al., 1993). Further discussion of this technology is beyond the scope of this chapter.

Imaging Analysis

The relationship between proximal musculoskeletal dysfunction and peripheral movement disorders mentioned earlier has been described and observed in many clinical situations. Careful attention to the scalene, sternocleidomastoid, pectoralis minor, and levator scapulae muscle groups is very important. Postural changes, including raised and forward-rolling shoulders as well as an anterior head carriage or forward-poking head posture, are common clinical observations. Mackinnon and Novack (1994) have recently drawn attention to posture in the etiology of cumulative trauma disorders.

Plain radiographs of the cervical spine may reveal degenerative changes at the appropriate levels that match the peripheral nerve impingement found commonly in the median and ulnar nerve distributions. The phenomenon of double-crush syndrome is often missed because of the failure to carefully link the proximal to the distal clinical findings.

Based on the cervical radiography results and nature of the proximal problem (which may be related to a sudden trauma or a continual repetitive motion), *magnetic resonance imaging* can be used to more clearly identify the nature and location of a structural abnormality at the level of the cervical spine and exiting nerve roots (e.g., at C5-6 and C6-7). Careful consideration must be given to the clinical implications of imaging results in prescribing appropriate clinical treatment and in predicting progress during the therapeutic exercise regimen.

THERAPEUTIC TECHNIQUES

Stretching Exercises to Restore Function of Damaged Tissue

A simplistic view of treatment would be to construct sets of exercises to stretch muscle-tendon units that appear to be tight or in spasm. However, this has proven to be unfruitful and often harmful from a clinical perspective. The key to designing a stretching exercise protocol lies in understanding all the biomechanical stresses on the functional unit, including the postural muscle imbalances that present themselves to the therapist. For example, by integrating with other clinical findings information about biomechanical effects of postural changes such as a forward-poking head posture and rounded, elevated shoulders, one can formulate a series of gentle stretching maneuvers to correct this frequently seen condition. The clinician should begin by helping the patient to both feel and see the nature of muscular imbalances in order to understand the relevance of frequent stretching and balancing exercises. The usefulness of video feedback to demonstrate postural abnormalities cannot be overemphasized.

Stretching exercises directed to the scapular stabilizers and the cervical flexors and rotators are extremely helpful in initially relieving pain that originates more proximally. Stretches of the flexors and extensors of the wrists and fingers are also important in relieving myofascial pain from common distal trigger points. If the stretching exercise routine is repeated in a correct and structured manner, a gradual restoration of normal movement pattern related to postural support and dynamic movement of the wrist and hand can be achieved (Pascarelli and Quilter, 1994).

Strengthening Exercises to Correct Postural Imbalances and Postinjury Deconditioning

The primary target muscle groups for strengthening and aerobic conditioning for an upper extremity work-related musculoskeletal disorder are the scapular stabilizers and muscles of cervical support. The cervical support muscle groups include the upper and lower fibers of the trapezius, with special emphasis on the lower trapezius area. Scapular stabilizers, including the levator scapulae, pectoralis minor, rhomboids, and serratus anterior, must be strengthened in a gradual fashion (Goldberg and Elliot 1994).

The scalene muscles are problematic, especially the scalenus medius. Tight fibrous muscle bands in the scalenus medius often interfere with control of the scapular stabilizers through the long thoracic nerve. This makes the process of muscle strengthening painful and tedious. The area of the pectoralis minor overriding the distal brachial plexus is problematic as well. Often one must wait for the effect of postural correction exercises to establish proper alignment before the process of strengthening and aerobic conditioning can progress.

Determination of the rate of progress of strengthening and aerobic conditioning is the key to correctly prescribing and predicting the time of return to work. The technique of surface EMG can be a useful adjunct. There is a regional fatigue after injury that requires considerable recovery time after exercises and work tasks. This recovery time can be determined by surface EMG and used to prescribe the amount of rest and stretching breaks. It should be monitored carefully using objective techniques—for example, by comparing the upper and lower trapezius muscles on both sides. This area of clinical applicability of surface EMG should be explored further.

Metabolic VO_2, or oxygen consumption, testing at baseline and throughout the course of an exercise program is extremely useful as well. This type of testing can also be used to monitor compliance, and ultimately predict outcome, especially in those patients who are slow to respond to therapeutic exercise.

Inflammation Management: Trigger Point Injections

The process of stretching and strengthening should be monitored extremely closely by the therapist. The number of repetitions and force as well as duration of the exercise cannot be prescribed according to a rigid formula but *must* be tailored according to clinical progress. When progress ceases, areas of deep and resistant trigger points can be injected with local anesthetic and corticosteroid.

These techniques of trigger point injection are well outlined in the text by Travell and Simons (1992). The areas especially resistant and often chronic are frequently trigger point complexes in the scalenes, levator scapulae, and pectoralis minor. By infiltrating these trigger points with anesthetic and stretching the therapeutically resistant areas, clinical progress can be resumed without delay.

The clinician must be very observant for sympathetic-mediated clinical signs such as changes in color or temperature and sweating. Obvious swelling of an extremity and intractable pain may signal the development of reflex sympathetic dystrophy and necessitate more invasive treatment: stellate ganglion block or intravenous infusion with substances such as guanethidine, phentolamine, or bretylium

(Hooshmand, 1993). This author has found bretylium to be particularly effective.

Passive Therapeutic Modalities

The usefulness of passive forms of treatment, such as ultrasound and ice, during the therapy process is restricted to superficial areas of regional inflammation. Local areas of tenosynovitis or nodule formation, especially in the flexor tendons of the fingers and extensors of the wrist and hand, may benefit from this type of treatment. However, there is a tendency for therapists to overutilize these types of passive modalities, and they are extremely limited in their therapeutic efficacy. Muscle disuse and atrophy sets in if there is not also a proper biomechanical analysis and prescription of appropriate exercises. Most therapeutic failures and delays in return to work are a direct result of misuse and overuse of passive modalities.

Acupuncture and Massage

Insertion of needles with or without electrical stimulation at specific acupuncture points can be helpful in resolving trigger point irritation and overcoming a myofascial pain referral pattern. The exact mechanism of pain relief with acupuncture is unknown but likely related to inhibition of the local pain response at the pain gate; possibly it is also centrally mediated from higher centers in the brain stem, as mentioned in Chapter 6 (Gunn et al., 1990).

Other therapeutic modalities include those of human touch, such as Swedish massage and Japanese shiatsu. These are passive methods of localizing areas of muscle spasm and a collection of trigger points. Areas of muscle that are resistant to stretching and strengthening exercises can be beneficially worked on with these mechanical techniques.

Medications

By the time of referral to a rehabilitation setting, patients have often had numerous medical assessments. Medications such as nonsteroidal anti-inflammatories and analgesics containing codeine are much *over*prescribed in this population. Also, because of the behavioral issues related to anxiety and depression, many patients referred are already on a mixture of mood-altering drugs and analgesics.

These medications in combination tend not only to mask the problems that are important to analyze in terms of symptoms and signs, but also to cloud the sensorium and impair the motivation of the individual. This makes it difficult for the worker to comply with the therapeutic exercise program. In general terms, it is advantageous to have a period of medication withdrawal at the beginning of the re-habilitation program so as to allow the therapist and patient to deal with the issues without pharmaceutical obfuscation.

Judicious prescription of short-term anti-inflammatories may help patients cope with pain brought on by the strengthening phase of rehabilitation, especially those with significant degenerative arthritis. In general, however, the use of analgesics for treatment of postexer-cise muscle aches only masks important clinical information required for the prescribing of force, repetition, and type of therapeutic exercise.

Relaxation Exercises

Much interest in recent years has focused on the area of mind-body medicine. The ability of individuals to control their own emotions and limbic function has been under recent investigation. This area of rapidly developing clinical science has been reviewed by Moyers (1993). Also, the management of the stress-related component of chronic musculoskeletal disorders is reviewed in Chapter 16 in this text. Self-taught exercise programs that can be learned on a commu-nity basis, such as tai chi, yoga, Feldenkrais, and Alexander tech-niques, are also very useful in this therapeutic area.

Educating, Enabling, and Empowering: Motivation and Compliance

During the therapy process, the need for compliance by the indi-vidual with recommendations given by therapists should not be un-derestimated. Throughout the administration of the therapy, all ther-apists and medical personnel must focus on this extremely important area of motivation and compliance. In some ways, the selection of patients who will comply with therapy may have more influence on outcome than the choice of therapeutic regimen prescribed. Once cli-nicians understand the crucial nature of this variable, they will be better able to control their outcome success rate. Unfortunately, the ability to identify those individuals who will comply versus those who will not comply has not become an exact science. For this reason, rehabilitation programs appear to be less effective than they might otherwise be.

Surgery

Various surgical procedures are available to treat certain work-related musculoskeletal disorders. These are primarily to relieve compression of a nerve or tendon, such as median nerve releases at the carpal tunnel, transposition of the ulnar nerve at the elbow, first rib resections, scalenotomies at the thoracic outlet, and cervical disc decompression at the spinal level. However, the role played by surgery in the treatment of chronic work-related injuries is small. Consequently, many hand surgeons, for example, have little interest in this area and, as discussed in Chapters 7 and 11, some doubt the physical efficacy of such procedures.

Clinical criteria for surgery are uncertain, and the decision to proceed with surgical decompression is indeed a difficult one. Much depends on one's therapeutic philosophy. Clear diagnostic information must point to the area of impingement of the peripheral nerve. The problem of a double or even multiple crush phenomenon affecting the peripheral nerve often fools clinicians and therapists. Much literature has discussed the controversial issue of unnecessary surgery. This is particularly true of thoracic outlet syndrome. However, Sanders and Haug (1991), in their text on thoracic outlet syndrome, have outlined the correct techniques of diagnosis and treatment for this nebulous condition and discuss the pros and cons of scalene muscle release versus transthoracic first rib resection. There is also clinical disagreement on the operative indications for carpal tunnel and ulnar nerve releases.

In summary, there must be clear electrodiagnostic indications that the peripheral nerve is in extreme distress before such decompression maneuvers are carried out. In clinical practice, the necessity for multiple decompressions will increase if the diagnostic discipline outlined early in this chapter is not carried out thoroughly. Furthermore, surgical intervention in a patient with severe psychological distress and chronic pain likely will save the peripheral nerve but do nothing for the chronic pain state.

THE QUESTION OF RETURN TO WORK

Ergonomic Modification

The return-to-work prescription is not only a science but an art form. Key ergonomic variables have been outlined in Chapter 4. From an ergonomic perspective, the problem facing clinicians as they prescribe return to work is the absence of accurate and reliable information concerning the specific job variables. It is insufficient to only specify the duration component. Often the information concerning force and repetition required by the job is absent, and job descriptions given by employers may be inaccurate or incomplete. Proper ergonomic assessment for each of the various facets of the job tasks is required, and for this a worksite visit by an ergonomist may be necessary. Once this information has been gathered on the jobs available, the clinician can then prescribe a return-to-work plan.[1] Often return to work is accomplished on a graduated basis whereby the employer offers some flexibility from an administrative point of view. Ideally there should be an occupational health nurse in the plant with whom the clinician can consult.

Timely and frequent follow-up of the injured worker during this phase is extremely important to allow problem solving and to reduce anxiety from the worker's point of view. With respect to the problem-solving process, the team has an opportunity to correct any offending ergonomic variable, often excessive force or faulty technique. Even the simple correction of posture and alignment during this phase via a proactive educational approach can often save the individual from a significant clinical relapse, or save time in the return-to-work phase of rehabilitation. Here the assistance of a nurse trained in occupational health on site at the workplace is a great asset. Chapter 14 discusses such a role in detail. Unfortunately, many factories do not have such a person on staff; however, if nurse consultants are available in the community, one can be hired on a part-time contract basis.

Controversial Aspects of the Return-to-Work Plan

The problem that confronts clinicians in occupational rehabilitation is the entity of chronic pain. Often by the time of referral to the clinical setting, chronic pain has already set in and is extremely resistant to the interventions outlined here. Overmedication, being away from the workplace for too long, being depressed, and losing the motivation to return to a workplace perceived to have been injurious are all factors that weigh heavily against therapeutic success. Psychological

---

[1]Recent advances in electronic technology allow transmission of data from the workplace shop floor to the rehabilitation setting. When such transmission is available, force and repetition information can be communicated through pictures and videotapes to allow more reliable and accurate prescription of these variables. However, this technology is frequently not available, and many clinicians asked to prescribe a return-to-work program may feel inadequately trained to use such technology.

and sociological factors are discussed elsewhere in this book and summarized in Chapter 17.

Depending on one's clinical philosophy, one can term this clinical situation either learned helplessness on the worker's part or, to some extent, a failure of occupational rehabilitation to correctly treat this clinical problem. Clinicians charged with the task of assessing this phenomenon offer a wide constellation of opinions that likely reflect their sources of funding rather than clinical truth (see Chapter 7). Careful attention to the previous clinical practice points will likely reduce the rising number of complaints and costs associated with chronic pain in the workplace.

What is striking about the assessment and treatment of chronic musculoskeletal work-related injuries is the complexity and importance of the pretherapy assessment. The implication is that, if one misses the diagnosis, one will make major errors in prescribing a therapy plan. Other clinicians believe that the key variables in management of these types of musculoskeletal disorders are not the diagnosis and the exercises, but the time of assessment and how the exercise regimen fits into the return-to-work plan. This is discussed at length in Chapter 12. Unfortunately, the time from first injury to return to work is often delayed in clinical practice. The prospect for return to work becomes extremely dismal after the 6-month mark in the natural history of the injury. At this point, prognosis for return to work is roughly 50 per cent. By the time a worker is off the job 2 years, the probability of return to work is less than 5 per cent. This explains strictly from a time management perspective why the disability statistics are so burdensome and medical treatment largely ineffective at this point.

Therefore, it is a clinical challenge to reduce the referral time from the workplace site of injury to the point of medical assessment and therapy intervention. The linkage between the workplace shop floor and rehabilitation clinic must be streamlined from a communications as well as an administrative perspective. The need to utilize computerized technology and efficient administration systems to speed up this process cannot be overstated, and this remains an area for future exploration.

REFERENCES

Goldberg L, Elliot DL: Exercise for Prevention and Treatment of Illness. Philadelphia, FA Davis, 1994.

Gunn CC, Sola AD, Loeser JD, et al: Dry-needling for chronic musculoskeletal pain syndromes—clinical observations. Acupuncture Sci Int J 1(2):9–15, 1990.

Hooshmand H: Chronic Pain—Reflex Sympathetic Dystrophy Prevention and Management. Boca Raton, FL, CRC Press Inc, 1993.

Mackinnon SE, Novack CB: Clinical commentary: Pathogenesis of cumulative trauma disorder. J Hand Surg 19A:873–883, 1994.

Moyers B: Healing and the Mind. New York, Doubleday, 1993.

Pascarelli E, Quilter D: Repetitive Strain Injury—A Computer User's Guide. New York, John Wiley & Sons, 1994.

Sanders RJ, Haug CE: Thoracic Outlet Syndrome—A Common Sequela of Neck Injuries. Philadelphia, JB Lippincott, 1991.

Skubick DL, Clasby R, Donaldson CCS, et al: Carpal tunnel syndrome as an expression of muscular dysfunction in the neck. J Occup Rehab 3(1):31–44, 1993.

Travell JG, Simons DG: Myofascial Pain and Dysfunction—The Trigger Point Manual. 2nd ed. Baltimore, Williams & Wilkins, 1992.

16

When Chronic Pain is the Problem

Brad Grunert _____

Pain is typically defined as the sensation accompanying the application of a noxious stimulus to the body. It is important to recognize, however, that the word "pain" is heavily laden emotionally and signifies both an affective and a physiologic state. The very terms we use to describe the noxious physiologic states are equally applicable to many of the negative emotional states that we experience. We routinely describe ourselves as experiencing pain when we are bereft of a loved one, as being hurt when others do something that contradicts our best interests, or as being injured as a result of others' disregard for our emotions. Pain, therefore, is intricately caught up with both physiologic processes and the emotional reactions to them.

MAJOR FACTORS INFLUENCING PERCEPTION AND MAINTENANCE OF PAIN

The first factor influencing pain perception is notions of *causality*. It is highly significant whether an individual views the causal factors resulting in pain as being accidental or intentional. Accidental factors are rarely accompanied by secondary emotional reactions such as malice or spite. In contrast, people who ascribe an intentional cause to a physiologic pain are much more likely to react with anger or depression. These factors can serve to diminish or to heighten the sense of pain an individual experiences in conjunction with a noxious stimulus.

A second major factor influencing pain perception stems from a *mechanistic viewpoint*. This viewpoint consists of a mechanical concept of the body and of the alleviation of pain. People who are highly mechanistic frequently believe that the part of their body that is injured should simply be replaced, much as one would replace a spark plug in a motor that was not functioning appropriately. They perceive physicians and medical personnel as having the same capabilities as the mechanic in the garage and, therefore, are highly incensed when a curative procedure is not performed for them. Individuals with this type of viewpoint have a significantly more difficult time coping with pain of a chronic nature than individuals not so disposed.

A final major factor that must be examined is the distinction between *discomfort and suffering* for the person experiencing pain. Discomfort signifies a virtually purely physiologic process. Misery, in comparison, is frequently accompanied by both primary and secondary gain and is heavily emotionally laden. Secondary gain is the well-understood concept of individuals deriving financial or other material benefit as a result of their ongoing suffering. Primary gain, however, is a less understood concept comprised of the emotional benefits that a person experiences as a result of pain and suffering. These may consist of increased attention from a loved one or detailed questioning by medical personnel. Such increased attention frequently fulfills unmet dependency needs in some individuals and results in them actually feeling better emotionally as a result of experiencing their pain and suffering. These factors are among the primary forces driving the maintenance of pain behavior of a chronic nature. Others factors are noted in Chapter 17 and illustrated in Figure 17–1.

EFFECT OF PAIN PERCEPTION
ON BEHAVIOR

Pain is an experience well known to virtually all of us. Our primary experiences with pain consist of acute pain. Acute pain is defined as pain that is of short duration. It can frequently be remediated by rest, which allows time for healing, with a subsequent return to function. We are all familiar with being lacerated, in which case we generally clean the wound, bandage the area for a few days, and allow the skin to repair itself. Following this recovery, we can again resume full activities utilizing the previously damaged portion of our body with no untoward effect.

Chronic pain differs significantly from the acute pain model. Chronic pain is by nature long term in duration. Long-term disuse, which frequently accompanies chronic pain, promotes a subsequent *loss of function* of the body part. Accompanying this loss of function are weakness, stiffness, and soreness when an attempt is made to use that part of the body. Individuals with chronic pain also experience a wide array of *affective reactions* to it. Frequently, they are angry over the fact that they have been incapacitated and that neither their physician nor anyone else can cure their condition. The fact that they have a chronic condition often results in worry and anxiety, which only heightens the perceptions of their discomfort. A final affective reaction, which develops over time, is depression. At this point, individuals feel hopeless about being able to control their own destiny and become overwhelmed by the fact that they need to face a chronic, ongoing discomfort.

The *behavioral effects* of chronic pain are reduced socialization and a reduced capacity for recreation and work. Chronic pain patients experience a sense of helplessness and a loss of direction for their own future. They describe themselves as feeling out of control and as being victims. There are additional difficulties with the fact that they have an "invisible injury" that cannot be seen by others and can only be manifested by behavior. Other individuals around the chronic pain patient frequently become annoyed with their repetitive complaints of pain and discomfort and begin to doubt the veracity of their reports. This results in further social isolation for the person experiencing chronic pain and increased depression and worry. Thus, a self-perpetuating cycle is established that becomes increasingly difficult to break out of over time.

Attributional theory, as proposed by Heider (1958), examines how individuals view the behavior of others and how they attribute causality to their observations. An individual observes the behavior of an "actor" and, as a result of this behavior, infers the causes that motivated it. Bem (1965, 1967) and others have done extensive research on the role of attributions. Attributional theory has a role in the development and maintenance of chronic pain behavior in several respects. The first of these is that observers view a chronic pain patient ("actor") and see reduced function and misery behaviors. As a result of this, they infer that the patient is experiencing acute discomfort. When these behaviors persist over a long period of time, observers may begin to doubt their original causal inference. Because these observers have had experience with the same acute model of pain that most chronic pain patients have experienced, when healing does not progress as they expect it to, they tend to look for alternate causes for the behavior, such as laziness, hypochondriasis, or the individual "beating the system." Once these *observer attributions* are formed, observers no longer provide the positive benefits of emotional support discussed previously and instead begin to isolate the individual even more. This frequently leads the patient to heighten pain complaints in order to legitimize them, and the vicious cycle continues. A major difficulty with most observers is that they have never experienced a chronically painful condition themselves. As a result, they are not able to conceptualize that an individual could experience pain over a long period of time. Therefore, one of the primary goals in the management of chronic pain is to reduce the pain behaviors that are present in order to reduce the misattributions formed by observers of the patient's behavior.

A second significant attributional factor that influences a person's coping with chronic pain are personal attributions. These *patient attributions* frequently deal with who or what is responsible for the ongoing discomfort that is being experienced. This has a great effect on the affective reactions that individuals experience. Metalsky et al. (1987) examined the role of attributions and depression. People who believe that they have no effect over the causes of their situation and therefore have no means of remediating it in the future experience greater depression than those who feel more empowered in dealing with the situation. Similar findings have been demonstrated by Grunert et al. (1992) for a hand-injured population. In this study of work-injured and non–work-injured individuals, there was a definite difference in attributional styles for the work-injured patients. Individuals with work injuries who entered the workers' compensation system believed that their employer's equipment was responsible for their injury in excess of 80 per cent of the time. Individuals injured in home accidents, however, believed that they were at fault for their injury over 70 per cent of the time. By feeling that one has control over the factors that led to the injury, it is easier to accept responsibility and to make changes that will prevent future injury. Such individuals feel in charge and are empowered by this. Those individuals who believe that they have no responsibility for what happened to them often resort to a victim mentality. They make attributions toward their employer of not caring or of being stupid or cheap. They also frequently think that their employer was malicious and was only concerned about production, viewing them as a disposable part of the operation. These types of attributions make it much more difficult for workers to return to that work environment because they are fearful and often believe they will continue to be misused in the future.

All of these factors have a significant impact on the rehabilitation and recovery of the person experiencing chronic pain. In order for effective rehabilitation to occur, such individuals need to undergo both an educational and a therapeutic process so that they can regain control over their lifestyle as well as the pain they encounter.

MANAGEMENT OF CHRONIC PAIN

Cognitive-Behavior Modification

The most effective models of pain management developed to date are heavily based on cognitive-behavior modification (Table 16–1). The basic premise of cognitive-behavior modification is that an event arises and then is filtered through the belief system of the individual experiencing it, resulting in a behavioral or emotional response to the event being produced. The key area of intervention, therefore, is in the belief system that mediates between the event and the behavioral/emotional response to it. Two of the primary models that have been developed to intervene are Albert Ellis' rational emotive therapy (RET) model (1962) and Donald Meichenbaum's stress inoculation training (SIT) model (1977).

In the RET model, patients are trained to actively refute beliefs that are irrational and damaging to them. In the case of chronic pain, such a belief may be "no one should suffer pain like this; my doctor should be able to take this away." Such a belief is maladaptive in several respects. First, it removes the responsibility for coping from the patient and places it on the physician and the rest of the medical system. Second, it promotes the idea that the patient is somehow being punished by experiencing a condition that no one else has ever suffered. The RET model would directly intervene in terms of altering both of these beliefs. It would emphasize the fact that the patient does have means at his or her disposal to effectively cope with chronic pain. It would also refute the second belief by stressing the fact that no one has a guarantee that they will not experience a chronic condition during their lifetime. By recognizing the fact that they have a

---

TABLE 16–1. Management Techniques for Chronic Pain

Cognitive-behavior modification
   Rational emotive therapy (RET)
   Stress inoculation training (SIT)
Development of coping skills
   Relaxation training
   Biofeedback to supplement relaxation
   Positive imagery
   Distraction
Goal setting that is
   Realistic
   Appropriately paced
Promoting realistic expectations

---

situation that is not punishing to them but, rather, is reflective of the circumstances of their life, and by recognizing that they can effectively intervene in this area, these individuals are empowered to take a more active role in coping with their chronic pain. Obviously, there are a wide variety of belief systems that maintain and interact with chronic pain, and these would need to be examined and addressed on a belief-by-belief basis.

Meichenbaum's SIT model develops the cognitive-behavioral perspective from a slightly different angle. The initial phase of SIT is to develop a model for what the patient is experiencing. It would be important in this model, therefore, that patients understand that chronic pain differs greatly from acute pain. Once this understanding is derived for the patient, then a plan of strategies for coping with chronic pain can be developed. A multitude of behavioral strategies, which will be discussed later, can be implemented into the development of a plan for coping. The individual then implements this plan and views the results of it. Strategies that were successful and beneficial in terms of coping with chronic pain are retained and those that were not beneficial are reworked or eliminated. New strategies are put in place and the individual again implements the plan and continues the process of refinement. The added benefit of this plan is that rewards are built into the plan so that, when patients attempt to implement the plan or successfully complete a particular circumstance of coping with chronic pain, they then reward themselves for having achieved this. This model is laid out in great detail in the book *Pain and Behavioral Medicine*, by Turk and colleagues (1983).

Development of Coping Skills

A variety of coping skills initially developed for patients with chronic low back pain (Grunert and Lynch, 1982) were later reformulated for use by patients with chronic upper extremity pain (Devine and Grunert, 1986). As with virtually all approaches to management of chronic pain, *relaxation training* forms an integral part of this. The goal of relaxation training is to teach skills that can be utilized in a variety of contexts to reduce physiologic arousal. The relaxation response has been found to be incompatible with the experience of pain and, therefore, allows an individual to experience a feeling of self-efficacy. Relaxation techniques can utilize autogenic induction, progressive relaxation, or hypnotic techniques. Depending on the individual, any of these may be the most effective means of inducing a relaxed state.

Biofeedback training is frequently used to supplement the relaxation response. This allows the individual to directly monitor physiologic activity in one or more ways. Thermal biofeedback of the extremities is a technique that has proved quite efficacious. In this approach, a thermistor is attached to the dorsal aspect of the long finger and the patient is taken through a relaxation exercise. Physiologic hyperactivity generally produces decreased blood flow to the extremities and, therefore, increased blood flow to the extremities is an indicator that physiologic hyperactivity is reducing. This is evidenced in biofeedback by heightened temperature of the digits. Allowing patients to see the progressive changes in temperature during the course of a relaxation induction greatly enhances their feelings of self-control and provides them with feedback that is rewarding to them.

Imagery is used, in conjunction with relaxation and biofeedback training, as an adjunctive form of treatment. The initial imagery exercises involve having individuals imagine themselves in a favorite place or at a favorite time in their life. This image is then conditioned to the relaxed state and can be called up in a variety of settings to provide relaxation and comfort to the body. Creating such an image allows the individual a place to which they can go to escape pain and provide themselves with a temporary reprieve from the effects of chronic pain. Some patients are able to progress to the point where they can actually imagine building barriers across their nervous systems that stop the transmission of the pain message to their brains or, alternately, to apply an image of cold or heat to the area that is affected, which again remediates some of the discomfort and pain. The use of imagery to deal with chronic pain is limited only by the patient and the therapist with whom he or she is working.

Distraction techniques have also been shown to be quite effective in chronic pain treatment protocols. The basic goal of distraction is to allow the individual to focus on stimuli that are not pain related. It is a common report among patients with chronic pain that, when they are engaged in activities that demand high levels of attention, their subjective experience of pain is reduced. Research has demonstrated that an individual can only process between five and nine pieces of information at a time. If the chronic pain patient is able to focus on five to nine non–pain-related pieces of information, there is no longer cognitive room to continue to process the ongoing message of chronic pain. When these patients are engaged in an activity, they can stop for a moment and briefly focus on their pain; it is as real and ever present as it always has been. However, when they are able to focus on the activities at hand, they are no longer aware of the discomfort that they are experiencing. Again, the goal of treatment is to demonstrate for patients in a very structured and effective manner the fact that they have control over their pain and do not need to experience it on an ongoing basis.

Goal Setting

Goal setting is another significant method of coping with chronic pain. Much of the time that patients have spent since the onset of their chronic pain has been focused on the losses in their lives that they have incurred. By focusing on a positive approach to goal setting, these individuals can be motivated to take a more proactive stance in their lives. However, they must come to understand that they cannot expect to do all of their usual activities and still achieve satisfaction from them. Chronic pain patients can be encouraged to keep a diary in which they monitor their behavior and establish goals that they are attempting to achieve, as well as evaluating the strategies that they have used to accomplish these. Patients can reward themselves, either through positive self-statements or through more material means, for achieving the goals that they have set. However, many of the goals are self-rewarding; accomplishing them and achieving the desired outcome is inherently satisfying and rewarding to these patients.

An important accompaniment to the goal-setting process is to work with chronic pain patients on *appropriate pacing*. Many of these individuals have high achievement needs and, as a result of this, drive themselves past what they ought really to be doing in order to achieve their goals. By focusing on breaking down tasks and activities into a variety of steps, such individuals can learn to pace themselves more effectively. Overdoing on one day will lead to markedly reduced ability to achieve on subsequent days. These patients must pace themselves and achieve on an ongoing basis so that they rarely experience the depression and despair that accompany the days following overexertion. Pacing allows them to get off the emotional roller coaster of feeling as if they are healing and achieving a lot one day and following this up with one or more days in which they are quite limited in their ability to participate in activities. Again, the goal is to have the individual take more personal control over his or her lifestyle and have confidence in the ability to do so.

Promoting Realistic Expectations

An equally important component to the entire process of coping with chronic pain is to teach patients that they should plan on experiencing exacerbations of their pain from time to time. They must be *realistic*. Despite the best laid plans and all of the coping strategies available to them, there will be times when they will either overexert themselves or run into activities in which they have not previously engaged that will lead to increased pain. Although they have a chronic pain condition, they can still experience short-term acute exacerbations of pain. These must be managed in much the same way that any acute pain would be—through brief periods of rest, icing, and elevation. By planning for exacerbations of their pain, chronic pain patients are able to circumvent the roller coaster of pain relief followed by heightened pain and accompanying depression. Again, this allows them to feel more in control of the situation and to cope with it in a more active manner, rather than being passive and relying on medical staff to do this for them.

CONCLUSION

The entire goal of pain management counseling is to put patients back in charge of their lives and of their behavior. This allows them to eliminate much of the "suffering" behavior that results in negative social feedback and increasing isolation. By *restoring a sense of control and personal efficacy*, patients are able to regrasp their own sense of the future and to engage in more goal-directed behavior. This allows them to maximize their recreational and work abilities as well as reduce their social isolation. Once chronic pain is accepted and is woven into the ongoing lifestyle of the individual experiencing it, it no longer is able to limit and control the activities of the individual to the extent it had initially.

REFERENCES

Bem DJ: An experimental analysis of self-persuasion. J Exp Soc Psychol 1: 199–218, 1965.

Bem DJ: Self-perception: An alternative interpretation of cognitive dissonance phenomena. Psychol Rev 74:183–200, 1967.

Devine CA, Grunert BK: Management of chronic pain in the upper extremities. Presented at the Ninth Annual Meeting of the American Society of Hand Therapists, New Orleans, 1986.

Ellis A: Reason and Emotion in Psychotherapy. New York, Lyle Stuart, 1962.

Grunert BK, Hargarten SW, Matloub HS, et al: Predictive value of psychological screening and acute hand injuries. J Hand Surg 17A:196–199, 1992.

Grunert BK, Lynch NT: Multidisciplinary management of chronic pain. *In* Chronic Pain Syndromes and Their Management. Chicago, American Medical Association, 1982, pp 7–10.

Heider F. The Psychology of Interpersonal Relations. New York, John Wiley & Sons, 1958.

Meichenbaum DH: Cognitive-Behavior Modification: An Integrative Approach. New York, Plenum Press, 1977.

Metalsky GI, Halberstadt LJ, Abramson LY: Vulnerability to depressive mood reactions: Toward a more powerful test of the diathesis-stress and causal mediation components of the reformulated theory of depression. J Pers Soc Psychol 52:386–393, 1987.

Turk D, Meichenbaum D, Genest M: Pain and Behavioral Medicine. New York, Guilford Press, 1983.

17

Mind, Body, Society, and the Workplace Environment

The production of this book has been motivated by a desire to meet the specific needs of individual injured workers. The problems they have require precise identification of the physical components as best we are clinically able, arrangement of therapy that recognizes the inseparable interaction of mind and body, and identification of risk factors at work with a view to prevention of such problems in the future. Chapter 7 has discussed the impact of societal values on the recognition of work-related injuries. The sociological battle that took place in Australia a decade ago is being fought in the United States today. We need now not only to consider the impact of society on the injured worker, but also to understand the worker's perception of injury, and what changes in the workplace environment might be desirable in the future.

FROM INDUSTRIAL REVOLUTION TO GLOBAL ECONOMY

Three centuries ago, life was hard and short; recreation was an unknown concept. Then came machines that revolutionized the world. A better life was forecast, but it was a long time coming. People fled from the farms, where they had spent long days in the sun-

269

shine, to the cities, where they lived in tenement houses and worked in factories overhung by smoke-filled skies. The machines chugged along as they did their work, but the machines could not do everything. Workers were required to do what machines could not. The machines were supposed to work for the people, but in fact the people worked for the machines, and the machines worked for their owners.

Circumstances slowly changed. Unions sprang up, giving power to the workers for the first time in history. The work week was gradually reduced from 70 hours to 40 or less, and we now have machines in the home that eliminate drudgery there. Recreation was invented, developed, and established as a human right. Now we have to work overtime to pay for household appliances, larger homes to put them in, and cars to take us to expensive recreational sites. Because of an explosion of knowledge, our children are now required to attend college or university in order to succeed in life. Educational costs add to our growing expenses. One job is not enough; we must have two.

Stress is now our constant companion. Employees are under stress. The health care practitioners who serve their needs are under stress. With lowering of trade barriers, even the employers are under stress. Stress is good—it increases productivity—but too much stress leads to illness.

When the industrial revolution came along, Britain could build an empire based on cheap raw materials, purchased in poverty-stricken countries, that could be converted into finished products manufactured in Britain. These products were purchased by the British at low cost, and even sold to the upper classes in poor countries, such as India, that had supplied the raw material. However, social values changed. Colonies in North America, India, Africa, and the Far East were given their freedom, only to emerge later as competitors on the international markets. The United States lacked an empire but had slaves to supply the raw materials. When slavery was abolished, the economy might have faltered, but more machines come to the rescue. Along with these came better means of transportation and communication. Because of these developments, it is now possible for countries such as Japan to threaten the economic status of the United States. What will happen when China, with all its masses of poorly paid workers, becomes truly industrialized? Stress. We will have to work harder to survive . . . or else lower our standard of living to the world average.

As our civilization "progressed," the workers became depersonalized, treated not as individuals but as pieces of the economic machine. After all, the human hand itself is a fantastic machine—a marvel of engineering. Coupled with built-in self-protective sensors and a computer-aided control system, it can do some things that no man-made machine can do. It even has a capacity for self repair, to a limited degree, and if damaged beyond repair, it can be replaced. Hands come two in a package but are very expensive. Sometimes they can be replaced at no cost if it can be established that the damage occurred elsewhere, or that the problem was really the fault of the manufacturer. The plan in some minds is to convince the world that injuries do not occur at work from overuse.

A battle for the mind is being waged, not with weapons but with words. Not everyone understands what the words mean, and those who claim to understand are changing the meanings. For example, the American Psychiatric Association (1994) has abolished the word "hysteria," largely, it seems, on the grounds that men also have this problem that was once erroneously related to the uterus. It is now called "conversion disorder" (Mai, 1995). Canadians had been calling musculoskeletal injuries that appear to be due to repetitive use at work "repetitive strain injuries" (RSI) on the grounds that these were *injuries* caused by repetitive strain. However, because the majority of Australians have concluded that RSI there was a form of psychoneurosis, Canadians are now starting to call RSIs "work-related musculoskeletal disorders." At present, the corresponding term used in the United States, "cumulative trauma disorder," is under attack (Weiland, 1996) for the same reason RSI was attacked in Australia. That reason is fear that there will be an epidemic of imagined problems that, through compensation costs, will ruin us all financially. Some go so far as to claim that no problem can ever arise from cumulative trauma. Others agree that such problems are possible, but state that, on the whole, repetitive motion promotes health (Nathan, 1995).

The issue here is not medical but political and economic. It is a battle fought within a society that was raised on television, and therefore contains many people who have difficulty at times distinguishing between fantasy and reality. The combatants in this battle, listed alphabetically, are advertising agencies, chiropractors, doctors, ergonomists, insurance agents, lawyers, manufacturers of therapeutic equipment, news media personnel, pharmaceutical companies, rehabilitation workers, therapists of all kinds, union leaders, and workers' compensation system employees. The arguments and the rationale for the positions of many of these groups are presented in Chapter 7.

Words are powerful; they are the building blocks of thought. Words put together well express ideas. Ideas repeated over and over will become established and believed to be facts—accepted as "common sense," whether there is a factual basis for them or not. Advertising agencies know this well. It is the basis of all propaganda . . . and of much of our education.

Words can also be dangerous, particularly if their meaning is misconstrued. For example, if a lumbar transverse process is fractured, this has the significance of a soft tissue injury. However, if the patient is told "one of the bones in your back is broken," there may then develop a fear of paralysis that converts a small problem into a life-long disability. Similarly, a herniated lumbar disc may be translated into an "exploded" disc. We need a diagnosis if it will influence treatment, but we must also be careful how we use such labels. Advantages and disadvantages of labeling must be carefully weighed before using them. For example, a diagnosis of fibromyalgia may put to an end a quest for diagnosis and treatment if accompanied by a program of pain management and a convincing argument against seeking a cure. However, such a label may become an added burden for someone who has already given up all hope.

DIFFERENTIATING ILLNESS FROM WELLNESS

Hadler (1993, pp. 16–33) offered some thought-provoking and useful insights into the concepts of illness and wellness by postulating that there are times when all of us feel "out-of-sorts" (see Table 17–1).

TABLE 17–1.   Components of the "Syndrome of Being Out-of-Sorts"*

Loss of the sense of well-being
  Decreased energy
  Easy fatiguability
  Bitemporal heaviness/achiness
  Inexplicable anxiousness
  Perception of a sleep debt
  Vigilance as to unusual symptoms
Musculoskeletal symptoms
  Diffuse achiness
  Disconcerting stiffness, often in the morning
  Sense of swelling, particularly about small joints
  Tenderness, often about the neck, shoulders, and low back
  Intermittent numbness of the hands and/or feet
Gastrointestinal symptoms
  Increased or decreased stool frequency
  Keen awareness of bowel function
Peculiar associations of well-being with external events
  Improvement with exercise
  Exacerbation with stress
  Exacerbation on gloomy, damp, and cold days

*Reprinted by permission from Hadler NM: Occupational Musculoskeletal Disorders. New York, Raven Press, 1993.

He stated that what individuals do about such symptoms, and how a medical practitioner approached about such symptoms handles the situation, will determine whether the individual becomes well or ill. It is in this kind of situation that labeling can become very dangerous. Hadler went on to draw striking parallels between the "syndrome of being out of sorts" (something we all feel from time to time), and fibromyalgia, irritable bowel syndrome, and chronic fatigue syndrome.

Although it is true that some injured workers and some physicians are guilty of exaggerating claims and finding problems where none exist, this is not true for most. While keeping an open mind to Hadler's views, we must remember the advice of Mahatma Gandhi: "Keep the windows of the mind open but don't allow yourself to be blown out the door" (from a sign in Varanasi airport, October 4, 1993).

Kleinman (1988) made the distinction between disease and illness in this way: A *disease* is a condition associated with structural or functional pathology, whereas an *illness* is the experience of having symptoms and of suffering from them. So a person can have, for example, tendinitis and the pathology associated with it and still be well. It is only when the individual perceives there is suffering because of a disease that that person becomes ill. The critical boundary is crossed from wellness to illness when the person with the pathology experiences sufficient discomfort to perceive there is an injury, and seeks confirmation of this from a health care practitioner. There are many factors influencing such perception, as illustrated in Figure 17–1. Because these factors run the gamut from physical and psychological through ergonomic to sociological, both in the workplace and beyond, it is clear that a team approach is needed both for diagnosis and management in many cases.

Factors in the Perception of Work-Related Injuries

Regarding the RSI epidemic in Australia, Spillane and Deves (1987) introduced the concept now echoed in the United States by Hadler (1993, pp. 1–4) that workers with pain *choose* to become patients with pain (or even compensation claimants with pain). However, Hopkins (1989) stated that "this account [of Spillane and Deves] fails to acknowledge that for significant numbers of RSI sufferers the pain is so intense that they do not perceive themselves as having any choice in the matter" (p. 253). This choice is based on a perception—a perception they have been injured. All those concerned with work-related injuries, on both sides of the battle, would like to prevent that

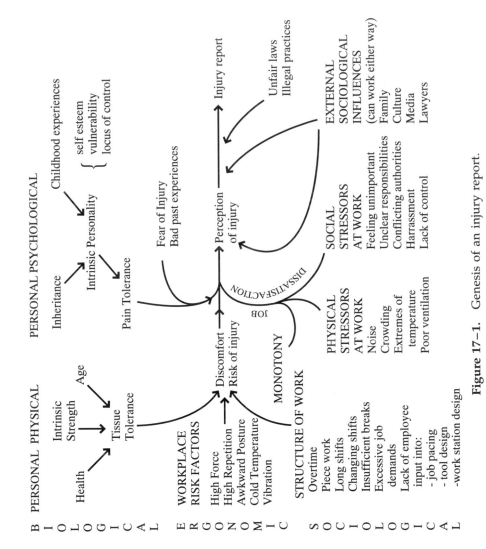

Figure 17–1. Genesis of an injury report.

choice from being made. To this end, we should unite and attempt to reduce, to the extent we can, the ergonomic, biologic (physical and psychologic), work organizational, and other sociological forces that combine to increase the perception of work injuries.

ERGONOMIC RISK FACTORS

Many ergonomic risk factors—job characteristics that, given enough exposure to them, are likely to lead to overuse injuries—have been identified. What "enough exposure" means has not been defined. Only a few epidemiologic studies have met the stringent criteria required to establish a probable causal relationship (Stock, 1991). Many other studies have shown particular overuse problems to be much more common in certain industries. In general, however, predictability of injury on the basis of risk factors alone is difficult, simply because there are other very important contributing factors that must be considered (Norman, 1994).

BIOLOGIC VARIABLES

Biologic variables must be considered, and the first of these is *personal physical characteristics*. Injury to any structure will occur if stress applied exceeds physical tolerance. Workers are not identical in strength. Obesity has also been cited as a risk factor (Nathan et al., 1992). Other health factors noted to contribute to specific conditions that can occur with industrial overuse include rheumatoid arthritis and various hormonal disturbances in carpal tunnel syndrome. Age and duration on the job should be obvious factors leading to injury, but this has not been shown to be the case. Possibly the reason for lack of correlation is the survivor factor. Those who are physically stronger, or who perhaps have developed less physically demanding ways of doing the job, remain working while those who just cannot handle the work leave voluntarily or as a result of injury. Seniority plays a role here and may allow workers of long standing to do less repetitive work and play a somewhat supervisory role. In this author's experience, when workers of many years are injured, it is often because the nature of the job had changed or the rate of production suddenly increased.

No work is free of discomfort. Whether this discomfort is perceived as pain attributable to an injury can depend on *psychological factors* that affect pain tolerance, both generally and specifically in relation to the particular job. General factors related to personality are the product of inheritance and of early childhood trauma and education—both nature and nurture. These *intrinsic personality traits* are very hard to modify in adults. Individuals with histories of being unable to control outcomes dating back to childhood may be particularly prone to become dysfunctional following a work-related accident or incident (Wall and Melzack, 1989). Specific factors include attitudes developed as a result of social interaction; these *psychological influences* can more readily be altered.

The most basic intrinsic personality characteristics are rooted in one's attitude toward self: Who am I? What am I worth? Am I vulnerable? Am I in control, or being controlled by others? *Self-worth* is based on one's intrinsic belief system coupled with a fair assessment of one's ability, in this context, at work. A good opinion about one's efficacy and worth has long been considered essential for psychological health (Maslow, 1968, pp. 152–155). With high self-esteem there is less tendency to focus on pain, knowing that, if this job does not suit, another can be obtained. If the pain intensifies, an injury report quickly follows. In contrast, a person with low self-esteem may fearfully view discomfort as the precursor to pain, and is likely to carry on without telling anyone until serious damage has been done. Inward focus on discomfort leads to perception of pain and of injury.

A *feeling of vulnerability* is probably the main determinant of an individual's pain threshold. This of course is in part related to self-worth and ability. It relates to one's perception of toughness (stoicism). It also relates to work organization (to be discussed later) in that someone who is a vital member of a team is less likely to worry about losing a job. However, anxiety about losing a job can easily translate discomfort into a pain that is perceived to represent injury. The anxiety about losing the job becomes a self-fulfilling prophecy. Anxiety in this sense should not be confused with a pathologic condition (i.e., an anxiety state). Here, anxiety means simply a heightened state of arousal relative to the particular situation. Anxiety per se (as a neurotic state) has been shown to be a poor predictor of occupational musculoskeletal pain (Ursin et al., 1988). Fear of injury may be reinforced by personal past experience and by such sociological factors as history of other workers suffering the same complaints, having a spouse on compensation, or alarming media reports.

Capacity for self-direction, or even the perception of such, has an influence on pain perception as well as being important in pain control. This relates not only to one's intrinsic sense of self but also to one's world view. Some people believe life is controlled by supernatural beings, by human political powers, by fate, or by events in a past life. Such people are "externally directed." When injured, they tend to be passive and depend on others to save them. A sense of helplessness possibly intensifies pain and certainly makes pain management far more difficult. Those who believe life is primarily influenced by their own actions are "internally directed" and are more likely to feel capable of rising above the problem. They are less likely to be fearful of injury and more likely to be tolerant of pain. The sense of being in control is an intrinsic personality trait related to a positive self-image. However, it can also be generated with respect to the particular job by a wise employer. While attempting to look at each area concerned with perception of injury in isolation, the health care practitioner must be aware that these all interrelate, as illustrated in Figure 17–2.

WORK ORGANIZATION FACTORS

Work organization has recently been the focus of attention for those seeking to develop better ways of understanding and preventing work-related injuries. Work organizational factors that increase risk of injury include overtime (whether forced or voluntary), long periods of work (e.g., 12-hour days), lack of sufficient rest breaks, piecework, lack of job rotation, and excessive job demands without the benefit of employee input. Just as those who do the job must be consulted when considering changes in design of tools and of the workstation, so also should they be consulted about all aspects of work organization. Where this is not essential for injury reduction, it will at least have an effect on injury perception. Shift work is another problem that increases both the risk of injury and the perception of it.

Workers who enjoy their work are less likely to perceive that discomfort or even pain represents injury. They are even reluctant to report injuries if they think they can manage without treatment. A

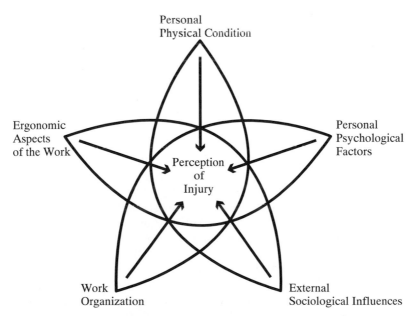

Figure 17–2. Interacting influences affecting perception of injury. *Arrows* indicate direction of increasing stress effect.

study by Bigos et al. (1991) indicates that workers who "hardly ever" enjoyed their job were 2.5 times more likely to report a back injury than were those who "almost always" enjoyed their work. Marras et al. (1993) reported similar findings. Dissatisfaction may occur for different reasons in different people. *Monotony* is characteristic of all repetitive work and may not always be remediable. However, job rotation that involves a variety of tasks will help relieve monotony at the same time as it reduces the physical stresses on the body parts being used.

Physical stressors in the workplace, such as noise, overcrowding, extremes of temperature, and poor ventilation, are obvious causes of dissatisfaction, but *social stresses* may be less apparent. Workers need to believe that they are each a vital part of an important team, that each is recognized as being valuable, and that their jobs are secure. For this reason, they should have enough work to do, the right tools to do that job, reasonable control over their rate of work, and a reasonable rate of pay. Sometimes work tension is inadvertently increased by having more than one immediate superior to satisfy. Job demands must be clear and free of conflict. It is unfortunate that ethnic and sexual harassment and/or discrimination also must be listed as sources of job dissatisfaction.

Employers expect employee loyalty. To deserve it, the annual picnic and sponsorship of a baseball team are just not enough. Each and every employee must be treated with respect by the employer and by all employer representatives. They must be treated as equal partners in the business. Loyalty works both ways. Many injured workers carry on at work in spite of pain and suffering because they feel themselves to be part of a family to which they have belonged for many years. This is particularly true in Japan, where such loyalty is reinforced by ethnic and work organizational characteristics. The sad story often heard on this side of the Pacific is that highly respected employees fall out of favor with management when they report an overuse musculoskeletal injury. If someone falls off a ladder and breaks a leg, everyone is sympathetic, but when someone who has done repetitive work for 28 years says "my arms are so sore I just can't continue," the employer and most of the co-workers turn and walk away. "Once I was the star of the production line," said one injured worker. "Now they don't want to know who I am." Rejection causes anger, the greatest potentiator of pain.

EXTERNAL SOCIOLOGICAL FACTORS

Other sociological influences in the home and in the wider community play key roles regarding injury perception. Injury perception may be reinforced by circumstances in a difficult *marital situation* (Waring, 1982). Sometimes a family quarrel is taken out on the employer and everyone around. Certainly any sense of having been abused outside the workplace is likely to make a person less tolerant of discomfort at work. Although many people have been accused of burying themselves in their work to escape a difficult home life, such work would never be the monotonous, repetitive type to be found in a factory. Rather, this kind of work could easily intensify the frustration and anger brought into the workplace from outside. People in such circumstances are already in a high state of arousal, ready to view anything bad as being worse than it really is.

When the spouse is on compensation, there is always a suspicion that examining the patient in the office only touches the tip of the iceberg. Is there a rivalry here for attention, a competition to see who is the more disabled and therefore incapable of doing the vacuuming? What games are being played at home, and how are the points to be scored? Perhaps the problem is not really at work at all. Perhaps pain, in this situation, is not a problem at work but rather the solution to a problem elsewhere.

Financial need plays an important role in reducing sensitivity to pain. Much has been made of pain enhancement to obtain a bigger pension. In the early stage, however, before an injury report is made, only fools would willingly give up their present salaries to go on compensation. It just does not pay enough. These workers are already getting a high rate of pay on the basis of high risk of injury, rather like army paratroopers who get extra pay as "danger money" because they routinely jump out of airplanes. The problem posed by high hourly rates of pay is that, when truly injured, a worker cannot afford to take another job that, having less risk, pays less money.

Where the compensation problem really becomes an issue is with the charlatan lawyers who wait like vultures outside factory gates and encourage workers to sue their employers on false claims. This does not happen where workers' compensation laws (as, for example, in Ontario) deny injured workers the right to sue (other than for negligence) in exchange for easy access to compensation benefits.

Reporting an injury can sometimes be difficult. Workers may be harassed by an employer in order to prevent reports being made that might force the particular employer to pay more money to the compensation agency. The animosity generated by employer harassment is harmful to both sides. The pain is intensified by this process, and the suffering prolonged, with more work time lost as a result. In some countries the laws promote reporting, whereas in others the laws discourage it. A favorite practice when fair legislation exists is to tempt the worker to apply for disability through an employer-sponsored private insurance policy. Then, if the worker is not fit for work when the insurance coverage expires, there is little chance that the compensation agency will accept a claim. This illegal practice is widespread.

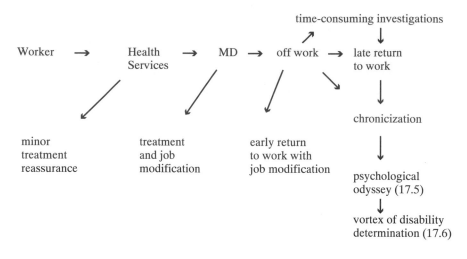

Figure 17–3. Potential results of work injury reporting.

The above discussion implies that injury requires time off, but this is not so for the majority of workers if appropriate intervention occurs at the worksite (see Chapter 14). Some may require only minor treatment and reassurance. However, the worker's complaint must be sympathetically managed and steps taken, if indicated, to prevent disability development. Job modification may be necessary, or referral to a physician may be required (see Fig. 17–3). The danger of chronicization if time off work is prolonged through extensive investigation and referral to specialists has been stressed in Chapter 12. Rarely, this may be necessary; often if it happens unnecessarily. The consequence in both cases is that the injured worker, now a compensation claimant, unfortunately enters what Hadler (1993) has aptly termed the vortex of disability determination.

THE PSYCHOLOGICAL ODYSSEY OF DOUBT AND DESPAIR

Serious injury has two major effects: it disrupts home life and causes absence from work. If the psychological consequences of work injury were anticipated in advance, most factories would be required to have warning signs about the dangers of overwork, in addition to those seen in Figure 17–4. Work rates would be regulated; piecework and overtime would be considered illegal, and desiring it immoral.

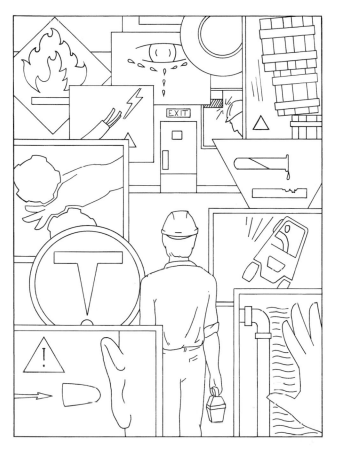

Figure 17–4. Surgeon General's warning: This work can be injurious to your health.

While the physical results of work injury can be very serious, the psychological effects can be much worse. For many people, their jobs define who they are. Without a job, life is meaningless. Very few are intrinsically idle and would like to live on government handouts . . . initially. The sad truth is that we are capable of adapting—so capable that we can physically survive on very little. What poverty destroys is not the body but the soul. A happy worker, proud of the fruit of labor, if disabled and out of work for a sufficient time, loses social contacts at work and becomes progressively depersonalized and de-humanized. This is the state to which military interrogators try to bring their victims. In such a state they will believe anything that is put into their minds: ideas about who is at fault, who they are, and how they should react, in this case, to their injuries. They are then quite vulnerable to suggestions by union representatives, the media, lawyer, doctors, and fellow workers.

Loss of self-esteem makes it easy to experience guilt. An injury to a small part of the body, such as the wrist, can prevent a worker from doing a job that depends on repetitive use of that part. However, when there is no obvious sign of injury, other workers and management may wonder if the complaint is genuine. The adverse climate that ensues can be a barrier to successful rehabilitation (Reid et al., 1991). Even the injured worker may wonder how such a small thing can cause such a great problem both at work and at home. Activities of daily living, recreation, family life, and marital relationships are all adversely affected. A typical reaction to this guilt is to blame someone else for the difficulty. Compensation received implies the worker is not guilty. If this is denied or considered inadequate, the message received by the worker is that the injury is not that significant. Consequent focusing on the problem by the injured party, coupled with a sense of rejection, intensifies the suffering and the symptoms become more widespread. A right wrist pain extends first to the elbow, later to the shoulder, and rarely may even involve the entire right half of the body. There may also be numbness and tingling that follows a nonanatomic pattern. This is *symptom magnification.*

So often clinicians hear the plea: "If only workers' comp would admit that I have been injured, I could get on with my life. I don't even want any compensation." It is not the monetary reward that such people seek but a recognition of who they are, that they are decent people and not malingerers. However, as long as there are people who do abuse the system—and there are a few out there—workers' compensation agents, employers, and other workers will be suspicious of someone who "just has a pain in the wrist and nothing to show for it." A careful examination with tests for legitimacy as described in Chapter 10 will establish what physical injuries have occurred. A just decision by all concerned will prevent the *need* for symptom magnification.

Compensation neurosis is a dubious diagnosis. Its existence as a clinical entity has never been proven (Kuch, 1993). A follow-up study of accident claims has demonstrated that compensation awards do not relieve symptoms (Tarsh and Royston, 1985). Rather, the adversarial nature of fighting for compensation produces considerable psychological distress. The interaction of disability, depression, and anxiety is represented in Figure 17–5. These emotional battle scars continue even after settlement (Guest and Drummond, 1992). Hadler (1993, pp. 258–262) described the process by which these emotional scars are obtained as the "vortex of disability determination." Hadler (p. 259) stated that the work of Crown (1978) suggests "psychologic

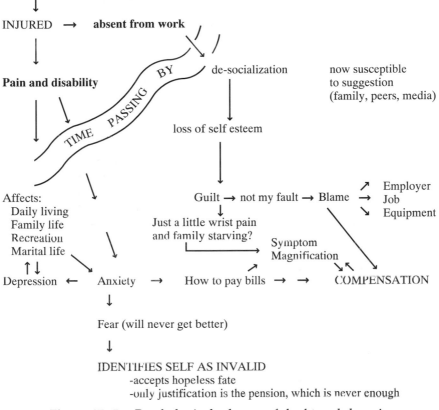

Figure 17–5. Psychological odyssey of doubt and despair.

aberration is acquired as a consequence of negotiating" their compensation for which these workers must repeatedly prove themselves disabled. Walker (1992) echoed the same sentiments, and suggested also that rewards without work being done and the uncontrollable dynamic characteristics of workers' compensation systems lead to the claimants learning helplessness. This downward path to learned helplessness is indeed a dizzying vortex wherein, as Hadler indicated, contrary advice is given (you are well, you are injured; you can go back to work, stay off another 3 months; take therapy and listen to what your body tells you, stop therapy and ignore your pain; hurt is not harm, don't overdo things; etc.). Although the injured worker's life may be likened to a vortex, as in Figure 17–6, it may also be compared to a roller coaster ride, with moments of temporary uplift (and hope) followed by even greater depression and despair.

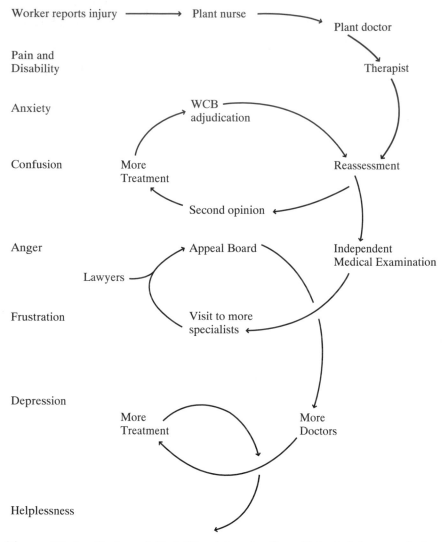

Figure 17–6. Vortex of disability determination. (Adapted by permission from Hadler N: Epidemiology of musculoskeletal illness. Presented at the Symposium on Cumulative Trauma Disorders II, American Association of Hand Surgery, Cincinnati, OH, August 11, 1995.)

Unfortunately, most of the advice given to the individual by "medical experts" is not based on objective evidence, such as a functional abilities evaluation. Rather, it is based on preconceived notions of the examiner, who in fact often has been selected because of the almost predictable nature of the report that will be produced. Such reports often reflect observer bias to a greater degree than the actual condition of the person being assessed. (For a discussion of such biases, see Chapter 7.) Through performing hundreds of noneconomic loss assessments for the workers' compensation system, this author has read so many of these reports that he can very often identify the examiner by the advice that is given regarding work capabilities and time for return to work. Such advice is many times given as a general statement that bears little relationship to the specific conditions of the particular individual examined. In effect, it may sometimes be a legislated policy statement rather than a prognosis regarding this individual.

TREATING THE WORKER AS AN ATHLETE

Comparisons have been made between workers and athletes with regard to the overuse nature of their injuries. However, workers and athletes differ in their goals and motivation, as mentioned in Chapter 2. The latest fad in treatment now is to treat injured workers "according to the sports medicine model," but is this really being done? Is it even possible, and, if possible, desirable? It would be interesting to speculate on what might happen if the workers were treated as athletes *before* they were injured. The supervisor, as coach, would be carefully monitoring the worker's performance, sending in a substitute when the worker is tired. There would be fostered a spirit of camaraderie. All would share joyfully in success, and be depressed when production targets are not met.

When an athlete sustains a mild injury, first aid is given on the field, simple preventative action is taken (e.g., taping of a sprained ankle to prevent repeated stress to injured ligaments), and the player resumes normal activity on the playing field. With a more severe injury, medical advice and/or investigations may be necessary. Sometimes the injury is sufficiently severe that it is clear from the outset the athlete may not be returning as a member of the team. This scenario is also seen in the workplace, and has been for a very long time.

When, following a severe injury, an injured athlete has achieved significant recovery, that athlete returns to the playing field to practice with the team under relatively controlled conditions. Even before this time, strengthening exercises are given that are done in the company of other injured athletes in an environment that focuses on athletic endeavors. The athlete never loses the feeling of being an athlete who belongs to a team. This same physical conditioning process is now being used in many places where work-hardening programs are given for injured workers. This is a large part of what is meant by treating the worker according to the sports medicine model, but this method, although a step in the right direction, is not working as well as it might. Problems exist that relate to attitudes and organization.

Although the worker may experience a sense of accomplishment when a job is well done, the obvious return for effort expended is monetary. Because workers are paid while off work, there is often a suspicion in the minds of employers, fellow workers, and many health care practitioners that the complaints may be exaggerated. There is therefore an *attitude of distrust* that increasingly pervades the atmosphere the longer the worker is away from work. Knowledge of this distrust creates anxiety, which compounds the psychological effects of injuries (Fig. 17–5), causing even greater pain and disability.

Because the injured worker's motivation may be automatically questioned, evaluation during the work-hardening program and subsequent return to work is often biased. If an injured worker cannot progress from one level to another according to a preset plan based on average expectations in a sports medicine setting, the worker is accused of "failing to cooperate." The same is true if the disability is due to a motor vehicle accident. However, if an athlete involved in a progressive strengthening program cannot progress to the next level, and in fact has more pain on attempting to, the policy in athletics is to drop back two levels and start again. *This* is rehabilitation according to the sports medicine model. What workers are given lacks this essential, biologically sound, and sensible system of stress modification according to tissue tolerance. When a worker is pushed to the limit, and the limit is respected, this worker is being treated as an athlete would be treated. *When pushed beyond the limit, the sports medicine model is not being applied.* This author's observation, and that of other sports medicine physicians who also treat injured workers, is that the sports medicine approach has rarely been applied in the management of injured workers. What has been aptly called a "work trial" is not the worker trying the suitability of the work, but rather the trial of the worker for failing to work.

We can do better. To begin with, the worker must be treated from the very outset as a valued member of the team. Plants that are large enough should have their own treatment and work-hardening facilities run in an empathetic and caring fashion. Smaller ones should have joint facilities run in cooperation with other companies, with government, or with both. In such cases, the injured workers should each day be required to show up at their plants to meet fellow team members and relate to them how hard they are working on their own rehabilitation. In Israel, compensation payment is contingent on the worker's attendance at work, however briefly. This avoids desocialization and maintains the sense of team membership.

Motivation should be assessed following injury, rather than assuming its absence. A clinical psychologist can be helpful in this regard. National sports teams carry psychologists on their roster. If we are to treat workers as atheletes, can we do less? The possibility of compensation being a motivation for not working is an issue based on laws that vary from state to state and country to country. Although it is fair and reasonable that an injured worker be compensated, the period of full compensation should have a defined term that is well known by all employees in advance of any claim. Workers need to be made aware of the fact that those who left on full compensation did not really do well in the end, as illustrated in Figures 17–5 and 17–6. Laws must be changed to prevent unethical lawyers from bleeding the system at the expense of injured workers and their employers.

Well before injuries occur, motivation must be strengthened in all workers. The more repetition and monotony is involved in the job, the more the workers need to take pride in their accomplishment—something positive to offset the negative. Athletes have pep talks to get them up for the task. Workers need the same. They need to realize that the company's success is their own success. This can be expressed in tangible ways by offering workers shares in the company at a subsidized rate, with bonus offerings to celebrate reaching company production goals. Any compensation for working overtime should be in the form of company shares. This would reduce the temptation and increase the sense of belonging.

When an injured worker returns to work, modified work must be made available. This may be temporary or even permanent. It should not be necessary to have a university degree in biology to understand that if a body structure (e.g., a tendon) can be damaged by a particularly stressful activity when it is normal, there is more chance of it being damaged when exposed to that same stress after it has already been injured. Yet doctors and other supposedly educated people repeatedly send injured workers back to the jobs that injured them. Apparently there is an assumption that the work injury was a chance happening. The fact is that *the work caused the injury*, and it will continue to cause injury until the injurious characteristics of that work are removed.

Again the problem is attitude. The employer often values the work more than the worker. The work must be done, and if this worker cannot do it, someone must be hired who can. The attitude of the union members is equally damaging. It is often the rigidity of union regulations that prevent an injured worker from moving into more suitable work, because the jobs that are less stressful are usually reserved for people with more seniority. This policy is not altogether a bad one. It allows older workers who are less able to handle the stress to continue working. However, its existence may force a younger in-

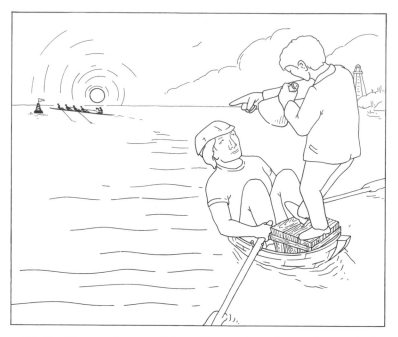

Figure 17–7. The worker as athlete: Even when the goals are similar, the atmosphere is quite different.

jured worker onto permanent compensation, so there must be some flexibility in the pursuit of this policy.

Treating the worker as an athlete has been talked about but not really achieved. A better analogy is seen in Figure 17–7. The athlete is treated with respect, but the worker with unfair suspicion in most cases. Where motivation is truly suspect, this should be assessed by a psychologist rather than attempting to do so physically in a manner analogous to asking someone to prove their innocence by walking over a bed of hot coals.

Compensation issues should not be prolonged. In addition to the financial cost of interminable disability determinations, there is the profound psychological cost (Fig. 17–6). The only beneficiaries are those who perform and record the result of these assessments. We need to define an end-point—for example, 2 years of adequate treatment, or 3 years maximum—at which a final assessment is made. Beyond this, there should be no reason to consider an appeal unless it can be shown that the proper evidence was not considered (in effect, a mistrial occurred). The effect of injury may be permanent, but the possibility that injury caused by work can continue to progress after the work has terminated should not be considered beyond a predetermined time.

BUILDING A HEALTHIER WORKPLACE ENVIRONMENT

Rather than focusing on injuries in the workplace, the compensation debate should concentrate on perception of injury. To the worker, it makes no difference whether there is really physical damage to the tissues or it merely feels as though there is. Those treating such workers and those working to prevent trauma must, of course, make the distinction. However, the worker with pain who has perceived this pain to represent an injury and filed an injury report has entered the vortex of disability determination, which could, if allowed, spiral the worker ever downward to a state of learned helplessness. The only beneficiaries of this process are the health care practitioners, claims assessors, and lawyers ... the very people for whom this book was written. We must, as Hadler (1993) suggested, stop this whole process now. With reference again to Figure 17–2, we can take steps to reduce injury perception in any one of five directions, or several at the same time.

Ergonomic Changes

Ergonomists have done much to identify characteristics of particular jobs that render them relatively harmful for most people in general, but, when it comes down to individual situations, what is harmful to one person may be well tolerated by another. The U.S. Occupational Safety and Health Administration is attempting to develop regulations with respect to rates of repetition, amounts of force, and the like that should be considered tolerable. A similar attempt to establish guidelines is underway in the Canadian province of British Columbia. This is an enormously difficult task because of the wide variability in individual response to the same work, and the wide variety of physical stressors present in the workplace. Standards have been developed in sports—for example, regarding hockey helmet design, by firing pucks at them and seeing which helmets would crack when subjected to stresses normally found in the game. A similar controlled study of computer keyboarding would require selection of a large number of people, dividing them, say, into three groups matched for height, weight, strength, and so forth, and assigning to each group a particular keystroke speed. Then, by assessing the number of cases of tendinitis at the end of a given period, we would have a reasonable idea of what constituted a dangerous rate of repetition for these workers. This kind of study is obviously not going to be done. In addition, because of the inability to control the many important variables in epidemiologic studies, it will be a long time before data are available that would allow useful guidelines to be developed.

In contrast to the ergonomists' attempts to fit the job to the worker, should we attempt to fit the worker to the job? It makes sense to suggest that, if a job requires a certain degree of muscular strength, cardiovascular endurance, flexibility, and so forth, we should not expose to risk a worker who is not physically fit enough to do the job. Much has been said about the advantages of exercise and fitness with regard to those already hired. As soon as the phrase "pre-employment screening" is mentioned, however, we enter the world of politics, where the playing field has never been level and likely never will be no matter how hard we try. It has been traditional to hire people who have the required education and skill in preference to those who do not meet these standards, but even this policy is now suspect in some quarters. Now we have other considerations: equal rights for disadvantaged groups based on ethnic origin, gender, and disability status. However, should the height requirement for an applicant to the police force be lower for women than for men? If height is important to do the job, is it not also important as a safety factor for the one hired? As we march to the tune of political correctness, are we putting the worker being hired at risk? The issue raised here is not one of morality but of safety. Here again, however, we do not really have any good data on which to base a case one way or the other.

Once hired, the employee's safety can be enhanced by such things as specific physical strengthening activity, training to do the job correctly and safely, and information about potential hazards of the job, how to avoid unnecessary stress, and *also* the acceptability of reporting concerns. The latter would be an opportunity for the employer to begin demonstrating concern for the employees, making them realize they are valued members of the team.

Past health records may provide information that would indicate whether there are significant risk factors in the new job for this worker. Workers must be able to confidentially reveal, for example, an old back injury, so that future risk of recurrence may be reduced. Is there sufficient trust in the employer-employee relationship to allow such a practice? Not at present.

Nonjob risk factors must also be discussed. Examples are the adverse effects of using the same muscles in a hobby (e.g., sewing) and the effect of nicotine as a source of muscle ischemia and a potentiator of pain. Will the employee accept such advice? Not likely, unless a genuine family atmosphere can be created in the workplace, and probably not even then.

Changes in Work Organization

Work organization must be the focus of attention for employers who are concerned with rising compensation costs. There is much that can be done to reduce the risk of injury, and the very act of so doing will counteract many personal psychological features that might otherwise reduce pain tolerance and increase perception of injury. For example, a worker with low self-esteem would feel less vulnerable and more secure through knowing the employer cares enough to encourage safety suggestions and implement them. Then, if the person who made such a suggestion were to be recognized by the employer, it is the employer's status that would rise. The responsibility of the employer goes well beyond the provisions of a safe workplace. There must be a friendly, enjoyable environment to which the worker wants to return each day.

It may seem financially more feasible to ask workers to work overtime, and pay them extra, than to hire more employees. This is because the expensive employee benefits package does not increase when employees are paid for overtime. The same applies to bonuses for increased production. Yet it is these very things, overtime and piecework, that add an extra burden to tissues on the brink of failure as a result of overuse. There are several questions here worthy of further study. Is it really more economical for the employer to pay overtime rates than to hire extra employees if we add to this the consequent cost of increased compensation expenses? Would the unions allow the elimination of overtime? Are the workers as well off as they imagine when offered this extra money in return for further physical abuse? What would be the political fallout if governments banned piecework, overtime, and long shifts?

Possibly the best initial approach would be to make workers more knowledgeable about these issues, and invite their input. If workers could be convinced of the risk of overuse injury, and made to understand the true financial consequences following injury, they might even be willing to accept a wage reduction for working less quickly. They would thus make a choice to focus on long-term employment rather than short-term financial gain. However, the psychological and sociological effects of soliciting input from workers are even more beneficial because each worker now feels important, and gains to some degree more control over the workplace environment. Just asking the worker's advice helps make the factory a more healthy place to be.

Karasek and Theorell (1990) published a demand-control-support model to explain the relationship between work, stress, and disease. They stated that it is the lower level workers, not the supervisors, who have more stress and stress-related health problems because it is not so much the job demands that generate stress but rather the "lack of control over how one meets the job's demands and how one uses one's skills." Social support reduces the effect of stress. Thus people who work alone are more vulnerable to stress and stress-related disease (Johnson and Hall, 1988). When workers find that management is supportive, stress is reduced and they are less likely to suffer stress-related problems.

What is most needed in the workplace is a sense of belonging and an increased sense of responsibility. When the job is boring and nobody cares about anything or anybody, the work is done merely for the paycheck. Job enrichment makes the job, not the pay, the focus of work. There must be more latitude given to the workers regarding when and how to apply the needed skills, as well as more control over time utilization and pacing, all within a framework of support and responsibility. The workers do not have the required skill to run the company, just as management lacks the skill and endurance to keep up with the machines, but they are members of the same team, like the offensive and defensive squads on a football team. Each has his or her own job to do, but they are all partners in production, working toward the same goals. There must be mutual respect and a shared sense of purpose. Then we will reduce not only the perception of injury but the number and severity of the injuries themselves.

CONCLUSION

This book began with the premise that workers can suffer chronic injury to the musculoskeletal and peripheral nervous systems through working at highly repetitive jobs. It ends with a brief exploration of the multifaceted aspects of etiology that go beyond the job and the individual to implicate society itself. In that microcosm of society, the workplace, we may find the reasons overuse injuries continue in spite of good ergonomic modifications.

More studies must be performed regarding specific aspects of the workplace environment. We must devise, implement, and assess innovative approaches to compensation, both for work done and following injury. For example, what would be the effect of company shares being given to workers on each anniversary of their employment, shares that could only be redeemed on retirement? Just as diagnosis and management require a team approach, so does this kind of research. In addition to sociologists, ergonomists, physicians, nurses, and therapists, there must be union members, economists, and business consultants on such teams. The implications of such studies would be far reaching, possibly involving the restructuring of unions and the radical reorganization of the way businesses function.

Prevention of chronic work-related injuries in a global economy can only be achieved with international cooperation. In North America, for example, if Mexicans do not have the same employee protection rights as Americans, Mexican employees will suffer injury while American employees face possible unemployment.

The universe is expanding. Human knowledge is increasing exponentially. However, the world is becoming a global village. As it does so, we are realizing more and more the interdependence of all things on each other. Ergonomic studies have indicated hazards in the workplace, but addressing only these issues is not enough. We must look beyond the purely mechanical aspects of injury prevention to consider the psychological as well as physical aspects of the persons injured, the way the work is structured, and the social environment in which the worker is situated. Work is not done in a vacuum. For most of us, it takes place at the center of our universe.

REFERENCES

American Psychiatric Association: Diagnostic and Statistical Manual of Mental Disorders, 4th ed. Washington, DC, American Psychiatric Association Press, 1994, pp 452–457.

Bigos SJ, Battie MC, Spendler DM, et al: A perspective study of work perceptions and psychosocial factors affecting the reporting of a back injury. Spine 16:1–6, 1991.

Crown S, Psychological aspects of low back pain. Rheumatol Rehabil 17: 114–124, 1978.

Guest GH, Drummond PD: Effects of compensation on emotional state and disability in chronic back pain. Pain 48:125–130, 1992.

Hadler NM: Occupational Musculoskeletal Disorders. New York, Raven Press, 1993.

Johnson JV, Hall EM: Job strain, workplace social support, and cardiovascular disease: A cross-sectional random sample of the Swedish working population. Am J Public Health 78:1336–1342, 1988.

Karasek R, Theorell T: Healthy Work: Stress, Productivity and the Reconstruction of Working Life. New York, Basic Books, 1990.

Kleinman A: The Illness Narratives: Suffering, Healing and the Human Condition, Chap 1. New York, Basic Books, 1988.

Kuch K: A psychiatric perspective on post-traumatic pair. Perspectives in Pain Management 2(3):3–6, 1993.

Mai FM: "Hysteria" in clinical neurology. Can J Neurol Sci 22:101–110, 1995.

Marras WS, Lavender SA, Leurgans SE, et al: The role of dynamic three-dimensional trunk motion in occupationally-related low back disorders: The effects of workplace factors, trunk position and trunk motion characteristics on risk of injury. Spine 18:617–628, 1993.

Maslow AM: Toward a Psychology of Being. New York, D. Van Nostrand Company, 1968.

Nathan PA: Pathophysiologic effects of inactivity. *In* Proceedings of the Symposium on Cumulative Trauma Disorders II, American Association for Hand Surgery, Cincinnati, OH, August 1995.

Nathan PA, Keniston RC, Meyers LD, et al: Obesity as a risk factor for slowing of sensory conduction of the median nerve: A cross-sectional and longitudinal study involving 428 workers. J Occup Med 34:379–383, 1992.

Norman RW: Occupational injury: Is it a psychosocial or biomechanical issue? *In* Proceedings of the 12th Triennial Congress of the International Ergonomics Association, Human Factors Association of Canada, Vol. I: International Perspectives on Ergonomics, McFadden, S, Innes L, Hill M (eds). Toronto, August 1994, pp 44–47.

Reid J, Ewan C, Lowry E: Pilgrimage of pain: The illness experiences of women with repetition strain injury and the search for credibility. Soc Sci Med 32:601–612, 1991.

Spillane R, Deves L: RSI: Pain, pretence or patienthood? J Ind Rel 29:41–48, 1987.

Stock SR: Workplace ergonomic factors and the development of musculoskeletal disorders of the neck and upper limbs: A meta-analysis. Am J Ind Med 19:87–107, 1991.

Tarsh MJ, Royston C: A follow-up study of accident neurosis. Br J Psychiatry 146:18–25, 1985.

Ursen H, Endresen IM, Ursin G: Psychological factors and self reports of muscle pain. Eur J Appl Physiol 57:282–290, 1988.

Walker JM: Injured worker helplessness: A critical relationship and systems level approach for intervention. J Occup Rehab 2:201–209, 1992.

Wall PD, Melzack R (eds): Textbook of Pain, 2nd ed. Edinburgh, Churchill Livingstone, 1989, p 1036.

Waring EM: Conjoint and marital therapy. *In* Roy R, Tunks E (eds): Chronic Pain: Psychosocial Factors in Rehabilitation. Baltimore, Williams & Wilkins, 1982, pp 151–165.

Weiland AJ: Repetitive strain injuries and cumulative trauma disorders. J Hand Surg 21A:337, 1996.

RECOMMENDED READING

Delvecchio MJ, Good PE, Brodwin PE, et al (eds): Pain as a Human Experience: An Anthropologic Perspective. Los Angeles, University of California Press, 1992.

Johnson JV, Johansson G (eds): The Psychosocial Work Environment: Work Organization, Democratization and Health. Amityville, NY, Baywood Publishing, 1991.

Karasek R, Theorell T: Healthy Work: Stress, Productivity and the Reconstruction of Working Life. New York, Basic Books, 1990.

APPENDICES _____

Appendix I

Minimum Clinical Criteria for Establishing a Provisional Diagnosis on First Assessment

A. Muscle/Tendon Disorders*

DISORDER	SYMPTOMS	EXAMINATION
Neck myalgia	Pain on one or both sides of neck increased by neck movement	Tender over paravertebral neck muscles
Trapezius myalgia	Pain on top of shoulder increased by shoulder elevation	Tender top of shoulder or medial border of scapula
Scapulothoracic pain syndrome[1]	Pain in scapular region increased by scapular movement	Tender over rib angles 2, 3, 4, 5, and/or 6
Rotator cuff tendinitis[2]	Pain in deltoid area or front of shoulder increased by glenohumeral movement	Rotator cuff tenderness, frozen shoulder excluded
Triceps tendinitis	Elbow pain increased by elbow movement	Tender triceps tendon
Arm myalgia	Pain in muscle(s) of arm	Tenderness in a specific muscle of the arm
Epicondylitis/tendinitis[3]	Pain localized to lateral or medial aspect of elbow	Tenderness of lateral or medial epicondyle, or of soft tissues attached for a distance of 1.5 cm
Forearm myalgia[4]	Pain in the proximal half of forearm (extensor or flexor aspect)	Tenderness in a specific muscle in the proximal half of the forearm (extensor or flexor aspect) more than 1.5 cm distal to the epicondyle
Wrist tendinitis	Pain on the extensor or flexor surface of wrist	Tenderness localized to specific tendons and not over bony prominences
Finger extensor tendinitis	Pain on dorsum of hand or wrist	Tenderness localized to specific tendons and not over bony prominences
Finger flexor tendinitis	Pain on the flexor aspect of hand or distal forearm	Pain on resisted finger flexion localized to area of tendon
Tenosynovitis (finger/thumb)	Clicking or catching of affected digit on movement; there may be pain or a lump in palm	Demonstration of these complaints, tenderness anterior to metacarpal of affected digit
Tenosynovitis, de Quervain's	Pain on radial aspect of wrist	Tenderness over first tendon compartment and positive Finkelstein's test
Intrinsic hand myalgia	Pain in muscles of hand	Tenderness in a specific muscle in hand

*Classification of severity of muscle/tendon problems:
Mild: above criteria met
Moderate: pain persists more than 2 hours after cessation of work but is gone after a night's sleep;
 OR tenderness plus pain on resisted activity if localized in an anatomically correct manner; OR: [1]Crepitation on circumduction of the shoulder, [2]Positive impingement test, [3]Positive Mills' test or reverse Mills' test (lateral or medial epicondylitis), [4]Pain localized to the muscle belly of the muscle being stressed during resisted activity.
Severe: pain not completely relieved by a night's sleep

298

B. Neuritis*

Disorder	Symptoms	Examination
Carpal tunnel syndrome	Numbness and/or tingling in thumb, index, and/or middle finger with particular wrist postures and/or at night	Positive Phalen's or carpal compression or lumbrical provocation test, or Tinel's sign present over median nerve at wrist
Thoracic outlet syndrome	Numbness and/or tingling on the postaxial border of upper limb	Positive modified Adson's test, 90 degrees' abduction and external rotation, hyperabduction, or shoulder brace test
Cervical outlet syndrome	Numbness and/or tingling on the preaxial border of upper limb	Tender scalene muscles with positive modified Adson's test
Cervical neuritis	Pain, numbness, or tingling following a dermatomal pattern in upper limb	Clinical evidence of intrinsic neck pathology together with nerve root sensory deficit
Lateral antebrachial neuritis	Lateral forearm pain, numbness, and tingling	Tenderness of coracobrachialis origin and reproduction of symptoms on palpation here or by resisted coracobrachialis activity
Pronator teres syndrome	Pain, numbness, and tingling in median nerve distribution distal to elbow	Tenderness of pronator teres or superficial finger flexor muscle, with tingling in median nerve distribution on resisted activation of same
Radial tunnel syndrome	Dorsal forearm pain aggravated by forearm rotation	Tender over supinator muscle, and pain on resisted supination
Cubital tunnel syndrome	Numbness and tingling distal to elbow in ulnar nerve distribution	Tender over ulnar nerve with positive Tinel's sign and/or elbow flexion test
Ulnar tunnel syndrome	Numbness and tingling in ulnar nerve distribution in hand distal to wrist	Positive Tinel's sign over ulnar nerve at wrist
Wartenberg's syndrome	Numbness and/or tingling in distribution of superficial radial nerve	Positive Tinel's sign on tapping over radial sensory nerve or positive provocative test
Digital neuritis	Numbness or tingling in fingers	Positive Tinel's sign on tapping over digital nerves

*Classification of severity of nerve problems: *Mild*: above criteria met; *Moderate*: if sensory loss on testing (does not apply to radial tunnel syndrome); *Severe*: if motor loss as well as sensory loss.

Adapted from Ranney D, Wells R., Moore A: Upper limb musculoskeletal disorders in highly repetitive industries: Precise anatomical physical findings. Ergonomics *38*: 1408–1423, 1995.

Appendix II

Intake Questionnaire and Assessment Profile

MEDICAL AND OCCUPATIONAL HISTORY

OCCUPATION: _____

1. Description of job task and equipment used: _____

2. Describe body position while working: _____

3. How long and often do you take breaks during your day? _____

4. What do you do during those breaks? _____

Background Information

1. List hobbies/interests and frequency of activity: _____

2. Change in lifestyle since incident:

	ACTIVITIES	
	Before	**After**
Work		
Leisure		
Domestic		

History of Incident

1. WHEN and HOW did the present problem begin? Please provide details.

_____
_____
_____
_____

Diagnosis?

Diagnostic testing (e.g., x-rays)? State date.

Treatment?

2. Since the incident . . . (please circle)
   Is your condition: stable   worse   better
   Are your symptoms: constant   periodic   occasional

3. On average, how long does your pain last? _____

4. What makes condition WORSE? _____

5. What makes condition BETTER? _____

6. Does a period of rest or activity influence your condition? Please specify.

_____

7. During the day does your condition change? (please circle)

   worse   better   same

8. Please indicate pain locations on diagram provided.

9. What does your pain feel like? Circle as many as you wish.

Burning	Numbing	Stabbing
Twisting	Pressure	Shooting
Stinging	Indescribable	Smarting
Aching	Throbbing	Dull
Cutting	Cramping	Vague
Pulling	Squeezing	Coldness
Tingling		

Other: _____

Specific Information

1. Do you experience any of the following? (Check any you have)
   _____ Ringing in your ears
   _____ Visual disturbances
   _____ Dizziness (feeling faint)
   _____ Nausea
   _____ Fainting
   _____ Vertigo (illusion of movement around you)
   _____ Headache
   _____ Numbness in the arms and hands

2. Do any of these reproduce your symptoms?
   _____ Coughing
   _____ Sneezing
   _____ Deep breathing
   _____ Maintained forward flexion (chin to chest)

Previous History

1. Describe any previous injuries and problems.

   _____
   _____
   _____
   _____
   _____
   _____

   Diagnoses?

   Diagnostic testing? State date.

   Treatment?

2. Please list names of previous physicians seen relating to the incident. Please list dates and enclose their reports about your condition.

Appendix III
Physical Assessment Forms

HAND, FOREARM, ELBOW ASSESSMENT FORM

NAME: _____   RIGHT   LEFT   Date: _____

HAND EXAMINATION

Deformity: No/Yes (specify)   Swelling: No/Yes (specify)

Color: Warmth: Capillary flow:

Sensory loss: No/Yes (specify)   Weakness; No/Yes (specify)

Tenderness: No/Yes (specify)

DIGITS

Active ROM: Full/Restricted   Open hole:

Max tip-to-palm distance: T   I   M   R   L

Crepitation   Triggering   Thumb abduction (deg.): _____

Degrees ROM (enter flexion in left box, extension in right box)

	Thumb		Index		Middle		Ring		Little	
	R	L	R	L	R	L	R	L	R	L
MP										
PIP										
DIP										

WRIST/FOREARM/ELBOW/ARM

Deformity: No/Yes (specify)   Swelling: No/Yes (specify)

Tenderness: No/Yes (if yes complete chart overleaf)

Active ROM: Full/Restricted

Degrees ROM

Wrist	R		L		Forearm/Elbow	R		L	
Flex/Ext					Pron/Supin				
RD/UD					Flex/Ext				

Passive ROM: Same/Different (specify):

Forearm muscle/tendon tenderness and pain on resistance (print M or T if muscle/tendon tender; circle if resisted pain; slash across circled M or T if incorrectly localized)

Right	Structure	Left	Right	Structure	Left	Right	Structure	Left
	Brach/Rad			Pronator			FDS Ind	
	Ext CRL			Flex CR			FDS Mid	
	Ext CRB			Palmaris			FDS Ring	
	Ext Dig.			Flex CU			Ext Pol L	
	Ext CU			Flex Pol L			Ext Pol B	
	Supinator			Flex Dig P			Abd Pol L	

Tenderness: Medial Epicondyle: R/L   **Lateral Epicondyle:** R/L

SPECIAL TESTS

Modified Phalen's: _____ Finkelstein's: _____ Allen's: _____

Tinel's (specify site): _____ Mod. Mills': _____

Carpal compression: _____ Elbow flexion: _____ Rev. Mills': _____

Lumbrical provoc: _____ Other (specify): _ _____ _____

Nerve palpation:

  Median: _____ Ulnar: _____ Radial: _____ _____

Investigations

DIAGNOSTIC SUMMARY

TREATMENT RECOMMENDED

_____

Signature

SHOULDER/NECK ASSESSMENT FORM

NAME: _____   RIGHT   LEFT   Date: _____

SHOULDER REGION
Visible deformity: No/Yes (specify) _____
Palpable abnormality: No/Yes (specify) _____

GLENOHUMERAL JOINT
Tenderness: No/Yes: Cor.   CA Lig   L.T.   Bic   G.T.
Other (specify):

Movement:
Scapulohumeral rhythm: Normal/Abnormal
Range of Motion:
  Active: Full/Restricted   Abduc   Flex   Ext   IR   ER
  Passive: Same/Greater
Resisted motion (circle if painful) and strength (underline if weak):
      Flexion / Extension / Int. Rot. / Ext. Rot. / Abduc. / Adduc.

Special Tests:
Painful arc: Absent/Present (specify range) _____

Impingement (Neer): Neg/Pos	Instability: Anteriorly Neg/Pos	
Impingement (Hawkins): Neg/Pos	Posteriorly Neg/Pos	
	Inferiorly Neg/Pos	
Supraspinatus: Neg/Pos	Biceps stress test: Neg/Pos	
Apprehension: Neg/Pos		

Other (specify):

Effect of Local Anesthetic in Subacromial Bursa:

PECTORAL GIRDLE (Describe any abnormalities)
Sternoclavicular joint: Acromioclavicular joint:

Clavicle: Scapula:

Coracoclavicular ligament: Scapulothoracic joint:

CERVICAL SPINE

Normal	Head Forward	Deviated: R/L
Lordosis: Inc./Dec.		Rotated: R/L

Tenderness

Midline:	0	1	2	3	4	5	6	7
R paravertebral:	0	1	2	3	4	5	6	7
L paravertebral:	0	1	2	3	4	5	6	7

Other (specify):

Movement: Normal   Mod. Adson test +90° AER

(If not, indicate range, circle if painful):   R: Neg/Pos   L: Neg/Pos

Flexion: _____ Extension: _____   Other TOS test (specify): _____

Rotation: R _____ L _____   R: Neg/Pos   L: Neg/Pos

Lat. Flexion: R _____ L _____   Facet test (ext. & rot.)

                                        R: Neg/Pos   L: Neg/Pos

NEUROLOGIC FUNCTION

Reflexes: B   Br   T   K   A   P

   L

   R

Sensation normal: Yes/No

Motor power normal: Yes/No

Specify if deficit:

INVESTIGATIONS

DIAGNOSTIC SUMMARY

TREATMENT RECOMMENDED

_____

                          Signature

SPINE EXAMINATION

NAME: _____   Date: _____

CERVICAL SPINE
Normal   Head Forward   Deviated: R/L
Lordosis: Inc./Dec.   Rotated: R/L

Tenderness

Midline:	0	1	2	3	4	5	6	7
R paravertebral:	0	1	2	3	4	5	6	7
L paravertebral:	0	1	2	3	4	5	6	7

Other (specify):

Movement: Normal   Mod. Adson test +90° AER
(If not, indicate range, circle if painful):   R: Neg/Pos   L: Neg/Pos
Flexion: _____ Extension: _____   Other TOS test (specify): _____
Rotation: R____ L____   R: Neg/Pos   L: Neg/Pos
Lat. Flexion: R____ L____   Facet test (ext. & rot.)
                                     R: Neg/Pos   L: Neg/Pos

THORACOLUMBAR SPINE
Shoulders shifted Left/Right: Standing: _____ cm   Seated: _____ cm
Pelvic tilt: No / L↓ / R↓   Leg lengths: L _____ R_____

THORACIC SPINE
Hyperkyphotic / Normal / Flat
Scoliosis: Convex L/R   Hump L/R

Tenderness

Midline:	1	2	3	4	5	6	7	8	9	10	11	12
R paravertebral:	1	2	3	4	5	6	7	8	9	10	11	12
L paravertebral:	1	2	3	4	5	6	7	8	9	10	11	12

LUMBAR SPINE
Hyperlordotic / Normal / Flat
Scoliosis: Convex L/R   Hump L/R

Tenderness

Midline:	12	1	2	3	4	5	Sacrum
R paravertebral:	12	1	2	3	4	5	Sacrum
L paravertebral:	12	1	2	3	4	5	Sacrum

SI joints: L   R   Upper Buttock: L   R
Trochanters: Piriformis: L   R
   L: post   sup   ant   lat
   R: post   sup   ant   lat
                                      Back of thigh: L   R

Movement: Normal

(If not, indicate range, circle if painful):

Flexion: _____ Extension: _____

Lat. Flexion: L _____ R _____

Rotation: L _____ R _____

SI JOINT

Movement: L   R

SI tests:

Schober test: 10 cm → ____ cm

Facet pain: L / R

Tests:	SLR	SST	FST
L			
R			

SYMPTOM MAGNIFICATION

Seated SLR

90° hip/knee: L / R

Hip rotation: L / R

Other tests:

NEUROLOGIC FUNCTION

Reflexes:	B	Br	T	K	A	P
L						
R						

Sensation normal: Yes/No

Motor power normal: Yes/No

Specify if deficit:

INVESTIGATIONS

DIAGNOSTIC SUMMARY

TREATMENT RECOMMENDED

_____

Signature

Appendix IV
Disability Assessment Forms

QUEBEC BACK PAIN DISABILITY SCALE

"Difficulty"

TODAY, do you find it difficult to perform the following activities because of your back? (Circle the number corresponding to the level of difficulty)

	Not difficult at all	Minimally difficult	Somewhat difficult	Fairly difficult	Very difficult	Unable to do
1 Get out of bed	0	1	2	3	4	5
2 Sleep through the night	0	1	2	3	4	5
3 Turn over in bed	0	1	2	3	4	5
4 Ride in a car	0	1	2	3	4	5
5 Stand up for 20–30 minutes	0	1	2	3	4	5
6 Sit in a chair for several hours	0	1	2	3	4	5
7 Climb one flight of stairs	0	1	2	3	4	5
8 Walk a few blocks (300–400 m)	0	1	2	3	4	5
9 Walk several miles	0	1	2	3	4	5
10 Reach up to high shelves	0	1	2	3	4	5
11 Throw a ball	0	1	2	3	4	5
12 Run one block (about 100 m)	0	1	2	3	4	5
13 Take food out of the fridge	0	1	2	3	4	5
14 Make your bed	0	1	2	3	4	5
15 Put on socks (pantyhose)	0	1	2	3	4	5
16 Bend over to clean the bathtub	0	1	2	3	4	5
17 Move a chair	0	1	2	3	4	5
18 Pull or push heavy doors	0	1	2	3	4	5
19 Carry 2 bags of groceries	0	1	2	3	4	5
20 Lift and carry a heavy suitcase	0	1	2	3	4	5

"Work Ability"

This questionnaire is about the way your back pain is affecting your ability to perform various work-related tasks and activities. *SUPPOSE* your job requires one of the activities listed below. We would like to know if you would be able or unable to perform these activities today. Please choose one response option for each activity (do not skip any activities), and circle the corresponding number.

Would you be able to work <u>TODAY if your job required any of the following</u> activities?

	Able	Probably able	Probably unable	Unable
1 Frequent lifting and carrying of light weights (5–10 lbs)	0	1	2	3
2 Frequent pulling and pushing with moderate strength	0	1	2	3
3 Frequent lifting and carrying with heavy weights (over 40 lbs)	0	1	2	3
4 Frequent twisting and stretching of your back	0	1	2	3
5 Frequent squatting & kneeling	0	1	2	3
6 Bending over or stooping for long periods of time	0	1	2	3
7 Standing up for periods of 20–30 minutes at a time	0	1	2	3
8 Standing up or walking continuously for several hours	0	1	2	3
9 Frequently walking up and down stairs	0	1	2	3
10 Sitting continuously for several hours	0	1	2	3

Reprinted by permission from Kopec JA, Esdaile JM, Abrahamowicz MJ: The Quebec Back Pain Disability Scale: Measurement properties. Spine 20:341–352, 1995.

OSWESTRY FUNCTIONAL ASSESSMENT QUESTIONNAIRE

Name: _____ Date: _____

Please read:

This questionnaire has been designed to give us information as to how your pain has affected your ability to manage in everyday life. Please answer every section, and mark in each section only the one statement that applies to you. We realize that you may consider that two of the statements in any one section relate to you, but please mark the box that most closely describes your problem.

Section 1—Pain Intensity

__ I can tolerate the pain without having to use pain killers.
__ The pain is bad, but I manage without pain killers.
__ Pain killers give complete relief from pain.
__ Pain killers give moderate relief from pain.
__ Pain killers give very little relief from pain.
__ Pain killers have no effect on the pain and I do not use them.

Section 2—Personal Care (Washing, Dressing, . . .)

__ I can look after myself normally without causing extra pain.
__ I can look after myself normally but it causes me extra pain.
__ It is painful to look after myself and I am slow and careful
__ I need some help but manage most of my personal care.
__ I need help every day in most aspects of self care.
__ I do not get dressed, wash with difficulty, and stay in bed.

Section 3—Lifting

__ I can lift heavy weights without extra pain.
__ I can lift heavy weights but it gives extra pain.
__ Pain prevents me from lifting heavy weights off the floor, but I can manage if they are conveniently positioned (e.g., on a table).
__ Pain prevents me from lifting heavy weights but I can manage light to medium weights if they are conveniently positioned.
__ I can only lift very light weights.
__ I cannot lift or carry anything at all.

Section 4—Walking

__ Pain does not prevent me from walking any distance.
__ Pain prevents me walking more than 1 mile.
__ Pain prevents me walking more than 1/2 mile.
__ Pain prevents me walking more than 1/4 mile.
__ I can only walk using a stick or crutches.
__ I am in bed most of the time and have to crawl to the toilet.

Section 5—Sitting

__ I can sit in any chair as long as I like.
__ I can only sit in my favorite chair as long as I like.
__ Pain prevents me sitting more than 1 hour.
__ Pain prevents me sitting more than 1/2 hour.
__ Pain prevents me sitting more than 10 minutes.
__ Pain prevents me sitting at all.

Section 6   Standing

___ I can stand as long as I want to without extra pain.
___ I can stand as long as I want, but it gives me extra pain.
___ Pain prevents me from standing for more than 1 hour.
___ Pain prevents me from standing for more than 30 minutes.
___ Pain prevents me from standing for more than 10 minutes.
___ Pain prevents me from standing at all.

Section 7—Sleeping

___ Pain does not prevent me from sleeping well.
___ I can sleep well only by using tablets.
___ Even when I take tablets I have less than 6 hours' sleep.
___ Even when I take tablets I have less than 4 hours' sleep.
___ Even when I take tablets I have less than 2 hours' sleep.
___ Pain prevents me from sleeping at all.

Section 8—Sex Life

___ My sex life is normal and causes no extra pain.
___ My sex life is normal but increases the degree of pain.
___ My sex life is nearly normal but is very painful.
___ My sex life is severely restricted by pain.
___ My sex life is nearly absent because of pain.
___ Pain prevents any sex at all.

Section 9—Social Life

___ My social life is normal and gives me no extra pain.
___ My social life is normal but increases the degree of pain.
___ Pain has no significant effect on my social life apart from my more
    energetic interests (e.g., dancing, etc.).
___ Pain has restricted my social life and I don't go out as often.
___ Pain has restricted my social life to my home.
    Pain prevents any social life at all.

Section 10—Traveling

___ I can travel anywhere without pain.
___ I can travel anywhere but it gives me extra pain.
___ Pain is bad but I can manage journeys over 2 hours.
___ Pain restricts me to journeys of less than 1 hour.
___ Pain restricts me to short necessary journeys under 30 mins.
___ Pain prevents me from traveling except to the doctor or home.

Scoring and Interpretation

Each section is scored out of a total possible score of 5. If the *first* statement is marked, the score for that section is 0. If the *last* statement is marked, the score for that section is 5.

The total score for the questionnaire is determined by:

$$\text{Total Score}/\text{Total Possible Score} \times 100 = \%$$
$$(\text{i.e., } 16/50 \times 100 = 32\%)$$

If one section is missed, or not applicable, the same formula may still be used.

RATINGS: Once a score is obtained, it can be interpreted using the following key:

0–20%: MINIMAL DISABILITY
This group can cope with most living activities. Usually no treatment is indicated, apart from advice on lifting, sitting posture, physical fitness, and diet. In this group, some patients have particular difficulty with sitting, and this may be important if their occupation is sedentary.

21–40%: MODERATE DISABILITY
This group experiences more pain and problems with lifting, sitting, and standing. Travel and social life are more difficult, and they may be off work. Personal care, sexual activity, and sleeping are grossly affected, and the back condition can usually be managed by conservative means.

41–60%: SEVERE DISABILITY
Pain* remains the main problem for this group of patients, but travel, personal care, social life, sexual activity, and sleep are also affected. These patients require detailed investigation.

61–80%: CRIPPLED
Pain impinges on all aspects of these patients' lives, both at home and at work. Positive intervention is required.

81–100%
These patients are either bed bound or exaggerating their symptoms. This can be evaluated by careful observation of the patient during the medical examination.

---

*This form was originally developed for assessment of the perceived disability due to back injury, but has been found useful for other injuries also.

Appendix V
Worksite Assessment Tools

ERGONOMIC ASSESSMENT FORM

Date Assessment Performed:
Job Location:
Job Description:
Assessment performed by:

Estimate the percentage of time the worker adopts each posture and indicate this percentage in the box beside the figure. Place a check mark beside the box if the worker holds this posture for more than 5 seconds at a time.

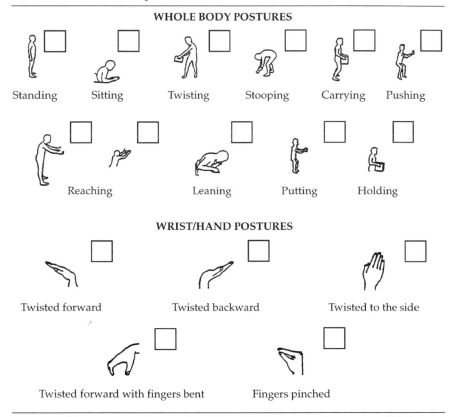

WHOLE BODY POSTURES

Standing   Sitting   Twisting   Stooping   Carrying   Pushing

Reaching   Leaning   Putting   Holding

WRIST/HAND POSTURES

Twisted forward   Twisted backward   Twisted to the side

Twisted forward with fingers bent   Fingers pinched

Reprinted by permission from Industrial Accident Prevention Association (IAPA) Canada from the Meat Processor's Workplace Inspection Kit.

JOB QUALIFICATION SHEET

Occupation Title	Location/Department	
Equipment Used	Supervisor	Date
1. Experience/Special Requirements	2. Education Requirements	
3. Physical Requirements	4. Working Conditions	

Complete items 3 & 4 as follows: 0—No Exposure; 1—Low Exposure; 2—Medium Exposure; 3—High Exposure
Describe all high exposures under Comments section

a. Balancing		n. Standing		CHEMICAL		PHYSICAL	
b. Crawling		o. Stooping		a. Dusts		k. Inside	
c. Climbing		p. Sitting		b. Liquids		l. Outside	
d. Feeling		q. Seeing		c. Mists, fumes		m. Temp.	
e. Handling		r. Color vision		d. Gases, vapors		n. Pressure	
f. Hearing		s. Depth perception		e. Odors		o. Noise	
g. Kneeling		t. Twisting		f. Special hazards		p. Humid	
h. Lifting		u. Use of right hand		BIOLOGICAL		q. Wet	
i. Pushing		v. Use of left hand		g. Fungi		r. Radiation	
j. Pulling		w. Use of both hands		h. Bacteria		s. Elevation	
k. Reaching		x. Walking		BIOMECHANICAL		t. Vibration	
l. Raising right arm		y. Working fast speed		i. Repetitiveness			
m. Raising left arm		z. Working fast speed		j. Fatigue			

COMMENTS:

SKILLS AND VOCATIONAL REQUIREMENTS

Position Title: _____ Hours worked/Day: _____

Status: ☐ Full Time   ☐ Part Time
          ☐ Student   ☐ Temporary   ☐ Rehab Placement

Department: _____ Section: _____

Supervisor: _____

Appropriate Season if Applicable: _____

For this position, the employee will require:

	YES	NO	(if YES, please explain)
Reading ability	☐	☐	_____
			_____
Writing ability	☐	☐	_____
			_____
Conversational ability	☐	☐	_____
Speaking	☐	☐	_____
Hearing	☐	☐	_____
			_____
			_____
Mathematical ability	☐	☐	_____
			_____
Clerical ability	☐	☐	_____
			_____
Mechanical aptitude	☐	☐	_____
			_____
Finger/hand dexterity			_____
Right	☐	☐	_____
Left	☐	☐	_____
Both	☐	☐	_____
Driver's license	☐	☐	_____
Use of vehicle	☐	☐	_____
			_____
Work experience,	☐	☐	_____
special training or			_____
skills			_____
Additional information	☐	☐	_____

Completed By: _____ Position: _____ Date: _____

PHYSICAL DEMANDS ANALYSIS CHECKLIST

Company				Date			
Department				Job title			
Task description							
Shift	Shift length			Time on task		Male/female	

Physical requirements					NO	YES	VERY
Precision, detailed, demanding work							
Repetitive work							
Light work							
Active work bending, lift, carrying, push, pulling, walking, standing							
Heavy work heavy manual work, loading/unloading, material handling							
Driving car/truck, forklift/manlift, other equipment							

Description	Y/N	Maximum weight	Average weight	Distance (cm)	Reps./cycle	Cycle duration	Cycles/shift
Lifting							
Lowering							
Pushing							
Rolling							
Carrying							
Fingering: right hand							
left hand							
Handling: right hand							
left hand							
Reaching: above chest							
below chest							
chest level							
Grip force: light							
medium							
maximum							
Grip type: pinch							
power							
Walking							
Climbing							
Twisting							
Kneeling							
Crouching							
Stooping							

Additional information:

Lifting/Lowering detail

Lift	————	Horizontal reach	————	Object size	————
Lower	————	Initial height	————	Assisted	————
Carrying	————	Final height	————	Handles	————
Combined	————	Distance	————	Twisting	————

Environment/Safety equipment

Hot	———————	Glasses/goggles	———————
Cold	———————	Ear plugs/muffs	———————
Inside work	———————	Gloves	———————
Outside work	———————	Respirator	———————
Wet	———————	Apron/coveralls	———————
Dry	———————	Safety shoes	———————

Workstation design

Is the orientation of the work layout adjustable? ————
Is the height of the work surface adjustable? ————
Is the location of handtools/equipment adjustable? ————
Can the operator sit while performing the task? ————
Are operators rotated on this task? ————

Quicklist

Body segment		Y/N	Body segment		Y/N
Shoulder	Reaching above chest		Low back	Repetitive twisting	
	Reaching behind back			Bending—knuckles to floor	
	Excessive arm extension			Bending—knuckles to knees	
	Excessive elbow elevation			Sit and/or stand	
	Excessive vibration		Neck	Poor neck posture	
	Extended static posture			Repetitive twisting	
	Excessive force			Repetitive flexion/extension	
Elbow	Repetitive rotation		Wrist	Repetitive rotation	
	Excessive force			Excessive force	
	Excessive vibration			Excessive vibration	
	Tool on balancer			Repetitive movement	
	Torque bar on tool			Using hand tool	

Additional information:

INDEX

Note: Page numbers in *italics* indicate illustrations; page numbers followed by t indicate tables.

Questionnaire(s) and inventory(ies)
(*Continued*)
  Oswestry Low Back Pain Disability
    Questionnaire, 206t, 316–318
  Pain Anxiety Symptoms Scale, 223t,
    223–224
  Quality of Life Questionnaire, 223t, 224
  Quebec Disability Scale, 207t, 314–315
  Sickness Impact Profile, Roland
    adaptation of, 206t
  Waddell, 207t
  Ways of Coping Questionnaire, 223t, 224

Radial nerve entrapment, 180–182, 183t
Radial tunnel syndrome, 170t
  clinical features of, 183t
  tests for, 181–182, 183t
Radiographic imaging, 249
Ragged red fiber(s), 27
Raphespinal pain pathway, 89, 91
Rational emotive therapy model, 263t,
    263–264
Raynaud's disease, 43t
Recovery time, duration of, 35
  frequency effect on, 50–51, 52
  from muscle fatigue, 22, 28, 35
  inadequate, 28
Referred pain, 19–20
  in legs, 139, 141, 141t
Relaxation training, in pain management,
    264
Repetitive strain injury (RSI), biopsy in, 10
  boredom and, 12
  epidemic. See *Epidemic.*
  epidemiologic studies of, 10–11
  in sports *vs.* industry, 11–12, 13t, 285–
    288, 288
  Koch's postulates of, 9–10
  media in, 1–2
  physiologic studies of, 11
  resolutions concerning, 2
  social movements and, 110–111
  terminology in, 1–3, 117–118, 271
Reporting of work-related injury, 231, 273,
    274
  consequences of, 280
  psychosocial stress and, 9, 279–280
Reproducibility of symptoms,
    implausibility and, 106
  work relatedness and, 71–73, 72–76, 75
Reticulospinal pain pathway, 89, 91
Return to work, 195, 205, 208–209, 209t–
    211t
  controversies in, 255–256
  ergonomic modification and, 254–255
  follow up after, 212
  initial occupational history and, 208
  job description and, 208

Return to work (*Continued*)
  job modification and, 239
  likelihood of, 256
  perception of incapacity to work in, 209,
    209t–211t, 212
Reversible fatigue syndrome, 2. See also
    Repetitive strain injury (RSI).
Rheumatoid arthritis, carpal tunnel
    syndrome and, 184
  of hand, 161–162
Rhomboid muscle, examination of, 126,
    127
Rib, second, as fibromyalgic tender point,
    142t
Roland adaptation of Sickness Impact
    Profile, 206t
Roos test, 173, 175
Rotator cuff tendinitis, characteristics of,
    129t
  diagnosis of, 132, 133–135, 298t
  physical examination in, 130, 132
RSI. See *Repetitive strain injury (RSI).*

Sacroiliac syndrome, 137t, 139
Saturday night paralysis, 170t
Scalene muscle, examination of, 126, 127
  exercises for, 250–251
Scalenus-anticus syndrome, 171
Scapula. See also *Cervical outlet syndrome.*
  examination of, 126, 127
Scapulothoracic pain syndrome, 129, 130
  diagnosis of, 298t
Schober's test, 136–137, 202, 203
Scoliosis, 201–202
Self-direction, capacity for, pain perception
    and, 276
Sensitization, interstitial potassium and, 19
  of free nerve endings, 19
Shear force(s), magnitude of, 28
Shoulder, anatomy of, 131
  assessment of, 308
  frozen, 135
  instability of, 134–135
  neuropathy in, 170t, 170–176
    musculocutaneous nerve entrapment
      as, 175–176
  pain in, capsular tears and, 133–135, 136
    impingement tests in, 132, 133–134
    in arc of motion, 135
    in pericapsulitis, 135
    in shoulder girdle, 128–129, 135–136
    in tendinitis, risk factors for, 42, 43t
    keyboard height and, 73
    neck injury and, 135–136
    risk factors for, 53, 54t
    scapulothoracic, 129, 130
    sources of, 129t
    work relatedness of, 72, 72